ABC OF THE
UPPER GASTROINTESTINAL

ABC OF THE UPPER GASTROINTESTINAL TRACT

Edited by

ROBERT PH LOGAN
*Senior Lecturer, Division of Gastroenterology,
University Hospital, Nottingham*

ADAM HARRIS
*Consultant Physician and Gastroenterologist,
Kent and Sussex Hospital, Tunbridge Wells*

JJ MISIEWICZ
*Honorary Consultant Physician and Honorary Joint Director,
Department of Gastroenterology and Nutrition,
Central Middlesex Hospital, London*

JH BARON
*Honorary Professorial Lecturer,
Mount Sinai School of Medicine, New York, USA*

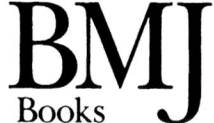

© BMJ Books 2002
BMJ Books is an imprint of the BMJ Publishing Group

All rights reserved. No part of this publication may be reproduced, stored in a retrieval system, or transmitted, in any form or by any means, electronic, mechanical, photocopying, recording and/or otherwise, without the prior written permission of the publishers.

First published in 2002
by BMJ Books, BMA House, Tavistock Square,
London WC1H 9JR

www.bmjbooks.com

British Library Cataloguing in Publication Data
A catalogue record for this book is available from the British Library

ISBN 0-7279-1266-6

Typeset by BMJ Electronic Production
Printed and bound in Spain by GraphyCems, Navarra

Cover image depicts *Helicobacter pylori* bacterium.
Coloured transmission electron micrograph (TEM) of a
section through a *Helicobacter pylori* bacterium.
With permission from Dr Linda Stannard, UCT/Science Photo Library

Contents

Contributors — vi

Foreword ROY POUNDER — vii

1 **Implications of dyspepsia for the NHS** — 1
RICHARD LOGAN *and* BRENDAN DELANEY

2 **Oesophagus: Heartburn** — 4
JOHN DE CAESTECKER

3 **Oesophagus: Atypical chest pain and motility disorders** — 8
JOHN BENNETT

4 **Dysphagia** — 12
WILLIAM OWEN

5 **Epidemiology and diagnosis of *Helicobacter pylori* infection** — 16
ROBERT PH LOGAN *and* MARJORIE M WALKER

6 **Pathophysiology of duodenal and gastric ulcer and gastric cancer** — 19
JOHN CALAM *and* JH BARON

7 **Management of *Helicobacter pylori* infection** — 22
ADAM HARRIS *and* JJ MISIEWICZ

8 **Indigestion and non-steroidal anti-inflammatory drugs** — 26
JM SEAGER *and* CJ HAWKEY

9 **Upper gastrointestinal haemorrhage** — 30
HELEN J DALLAL *and* KR PALMER

10 **Indigestion: When is it functional?** — 33
NICHOLAS J TALLEY, NGHI PHUNG *and* JAMSHID S KALANTAR

11 **Upper abdominal pain: Gall bladder** — 37
CD JOHNSON

12 **Cancer of the stomach and pancreas** — 41
MATTHEW J BOWLES *and* IRVING S BENJAMIN

13 **Anorexia, nausea, vomiting, and pain** — 45
RC SPILLER

Index — 49

Contributors

JH Baron
Honorary Professorial Lecturer, Mount Sinai School of Medicine, New York, USA

Irving S Benjamin
Professor of Surgery, Guy's, King's and St Thomas's School of Medicine, Kings College, London

John Bennett
Treasurer, Royal College of Physicians, London

Matthew J Bowles
Consultant Liver Transplant and General Surgeon, King's College Hospital, London

John de Caestecker
Consultant Gastroenterologist, Glenfield Hospital NHS Trust, Leicester

John Calam
Professor of Gastroenterology, Imperial College School of Medicine, London

Helen J Dallal
Specialist Registrar, Royal Aberdeen Infirmary, Aberdeen

Brendan Delaney
Reader in Primary Care and General Practice, University of Birmingham, Birmingham

Adam Harris
Consultant Physician and Gastroenterologist, Kent and Sussex Hospital, Tunbridge Wells

CJ Hawkey
Professor of Gastroenterology, University Hospital, Nottingham

CD Johnson
Reader in Surgery, University Surgical Unit, Southampton General Hospital, Southampton

Jamshid S Kalantar
Staff Specialist in Gastroenterology, Department of Medicine, University of Sydney, Nepean Hospital, Penrith, Australia

Richard Logan
Professor of Clinical Epidemiology, University Hospital, Nottingham

Robert PH Logan
Senior Lecturer, Division of Gastroenterology, University Hospital, Nottingham

JJ Misiewicz
Honorary Consultant Physician and Honorary Joint Director of the Department of Gastroenterology and Nutrition, Central Middlesex Hospital, London

William Owen
Consultant Surgeon, Guy's and St Thomas's Hospital Trust, London

KR Palmer
Consultant Gastroenterologist, Western General Hospital, Edinburgh

Nghi Phung
Gastroenterologist, Department of Medicine, University of Sydney, Nepean Hospital, Penrith, Australia

RC Spiller
Professor of Gastroenterology, University of Nottingham

JM Seager
Research Pharmacist, Division of Gastroenterology, University Hospital, Nottingham

Nicholas J Talley
Professor of Medicine, Department of Medicine, University of Sydney, Nepean Hospital, Penrith, Australia

Marjorie M Walker
Senior Lecturer, Department of Histopathology, Imperial College, London

Foreword

Robert Logan, Adam Harris, George Misiewicz and Hugh Baron, the Editors of *ABC of the Upper Gastrointestinal Tract*, are all closely associated with Sir Francis Avery Jones and the Central Middlesex Hospital. Thirty years ago this month I started with Sir Francis as his last Medical Registrar, and that is why I have been invited to write this Foreword.

Sir Francis was famous for saving the lives of pre-war patients with bleeding peptic ulcers by offering food and fluid, rather than starvation. With Sir Richard Doll, he introduced controlled clinical trials for peptic ulcer disease (indeed for all diseases, in due course), showing that carbenoxolone was better than placebo for gastric ulcer healing. He relied upon barium meals to diagnose ulcers and cancer.

How would Sir Francis recognise this excellent collection of 13 articles about the upper gastrointestinal tract? Well, a lot has changed because of the three factors that damage this part of the human body – acid, *Helicobacter pylori* and non-steroidal anti-inflammatory drugs. Our ability to image this part of the body is another big development. Finally, having thought that we'd made surgeons redundant, they have staged a comeback.

For 25 years we have been able to decrease acid secretion moderately with histamine H_2 receptor antagonists, and for 15 years we have had powerful control using proton pump inhibitors. We thought that this could deal with everything acidic, albeit with the need for indefinite maintenance treatment. But in 1981 Warren and Marshall identified, with typical Australian confidence, *H pylori*. Eradication was the new excitement – mostly curing duodenal ulceration, but leaving a "healthy" stomach with plentiful acid secretion, and the liability for acid reflux. So Sir Francis would be missing peptic ulceration, and would be more concerned about reflux, Barrett's oesophagus, and oesophageal cancer. Our ageing population welcomed the pain relief and mobility achieved by non-steroidal anti-inflammatory drugs – only to be troubled by peptic ulcers that were often silent until they haemorrhaged or perforated. The best of times, the worst of times …

The improvements in our ability to investigate this area have been breathtaking: endoscopy, ultrasound, retrograde cholangiopancreatography, computerised tomography, magnetic resonance cholangiopancreatography, endoscopic ultrasound, ^{13}C-urea breath testing, oesophageal manometry, and pH profiles. Organic disease can be excluded by exhaustive investigations, and functional disorders are the new challenge.

Finally, the development of minimally invasive surgery leads the surgical renaissance. No longer gastric resections for chronic peptic ulcer disease – now laparoscopic cholecystectomy for gallstones identified by ultrasound, or fundoplication for the acid reflux that now damages the oesophagus.

This explains why I welcome this collection of articles about the upper gastrointestinal tract – it is an amazing story of rapid advance and excitement, of genuine medical and surgical achievement, with real improvement in the quality of life for many of our patients. The Editors and authors of *ABC of the Upper Gastrointestinal Tract* have created a book that would have intrigued Sir Francis.

Roy Pounder
Royal Free Hospital, London

1 Implications of dyspepsia for the NHS

Richard Logan, Brendan Delaney

There is no precise definition of dyspepsia. It can be defined pragmatically as upper abdominal or retrosternal pain, with or without other symptoms thought to be arising from the upper gastrointestinal tract—which is the approach that has been generally adopted by epidemiological studies.

It has been suggested that dyspeptic symptoms can be categorised as ulcer-like, reflux-like, and dysmotility-like as a guide to the underlying cause. These groups, however, overlap considerably, with mixed patterns being common. Symptom patterns are not strong predictors of underlying disease. Recently it has been proposed that if heartburn or acid regurgitation are the dominant symptoms then these are sufficiently accurate predictors of gastro-oesophageal reflux to make a safe and accurate diagnosis (see next article). Fewer than a fifth of sufferers have this symptom pattern, and the predictive accuracy needs confirmation.

Prevalence

Dyspepsia is common: in a recent UK survey 40% of adults reported having had one or more dyspeptic symptoms in the previous year, and about a half described these as being moderate to severe. Of this group, more than half were taking drugs for dyspepsia (40% of which were prescribed) and 22% had seen their general practitioner about dyspepsia in the previous year. Thus, 9% of all those interviewed reported consulting their doctor about dyspepsia in the previous year.

Most dyspeptic patients have no clinically significant abnormalities on investigation. Up to 20% may have endoscopic reflux oesophagitis, and 15-20% may have peptic ulcer disease, including duodenitis. A declining proportion, currently around 2%, will have a gastric or oesophageal cancer, with other "alarm" symptoms such as dysphagia or weight loss usually being present.

Whether dyspepsia is becoming more common is unclear, but general practice consultations for non-ulcer dyspepsia have been increasing. In contrast, morbidity and mortality resulting from peptic ulcer disease is declining; mortality from oesophageal cancer has now overtaken mortality from gastric cancer, which has declined steeply over the past 50 years.

Cost to the NHS

The management of these patients has a considerable impact on the NHS. At any one time up to 4% of the population are thought to be taking prescribed drugs for dyspepsia. In the past few years the costs of these prescriptions have risen dramatically and now account for over 10% of drug expenditure in primary care (471m in 1999 in England and Wales), although this may now have peaked.

Investigation is also costly. The number of upper gastroscopies performed each year in the United Kingdom has been steadily increasing and was thought to be over 450 000 in 1996, a little over one endoscopy for every 100 adults in England and Wales. Endoscopy has been estimated to cost £80-£450 per procedure depending on the hospital (NHS Reference costs 1998). In addition, assessment of dyspepsia and abdominal pain is one of the commonest reasons for referral to hospital.

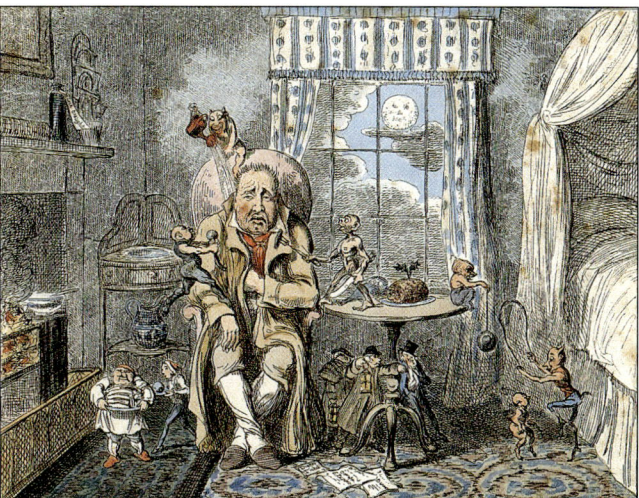

Figure 1.1 Dyspepsia is not new and has been known throughout history (*Indigestion* by Cruickshank (1792-1872))

Box 1.1 "Alarm" symptoms in patients with dyspepsia suggesting possibility of malignant disease

- **A**naemia
- **L**oss of weight
- **A**norexia
- **R**ecent onset of progressive symptoms (<3 months)
- **M**elaena or haematemesis
- **D**ysphagia

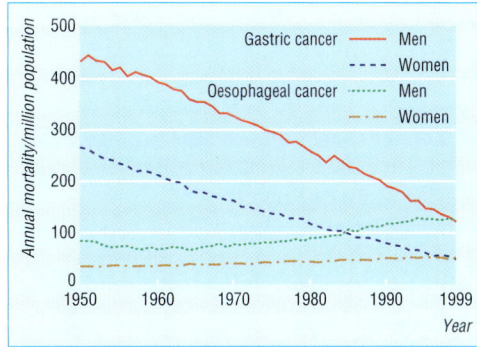

Figure 1.2 Mortality from gastric and oesophageal cancer in England and Wales 1950-99

Table 1.1 Patients consulting with upper gastrointestinal disorders in general practitioner morbidity surveys

	No of patients (per 10 000/year)		
Condition (ICD code)	**1981-2**	**1991-2**	**Change**
Non-ulcer dyspepsia:	178	330	85%
Oesophagus (530)	24	103	
Gastritis or duodenitis (535)	27	74	
Other disorders (536)	127	153	
Peptic ulcer (531-534)	57	52	−9%
All disorders	720	866	20%

ABC of the Upper Gastrointestinal Tract

To these costs one might also add the costs of managing complications such as gastrointestinal bleeding from peptic ulceration and oesophagitis.

Managing dyspepsia in primary care

Why do patients consult with dyspepsia?
According to the health belief model, the decision to consult a general practitioner is determined by a person's perception of the likelihood of serious disease and the potential for cure.

Five factors are thought to influence whether a patient consults a doctor: how the patient perceives the problem, how the patient's peers perceive the problem, the availability of medical care, the availability of non-medical treatments, and whether the patient can afford treatment. Other triggers—such as an interpersonal crisis; interference with personal relationships, work, or physical functioning; sanctioning; and setting of external time criteria—are required to force a medicalisation of the symptoms before they are perceived as illness.

Qualitative studies have shown that patients with dyspepsia are concerned with finding causal relations between life events and their symptoms. "Stomach disease" is most commonly linked to stress and worry. No difference has been found between people who consult a doctor about their dyspepsia and those who do not in the frequency or subjective severity of their symptoms, but those who do consult have significantly more life events. People consulting with dyspepsia are more likely to believe that their symptoms are due to serious illness, heart disease, ulcers, or cancer in particular. The challenge for general practitioners is to maximise detection of serious and treatable conditions while minimising the cost and adverse effects of investigation.

Strategies for managing dyspepsia in primary care

Initial empiric treatment with antacids or anti-secretory drugs
A period of empiric treatment with antacids or H_2 receptor antagonists has been the traditional strategy for managing patients with dyspepsia first consulting their doctor. This strategy recognises that most patients' symptoms are episodic and remit spontaneously and that the risk of peptic ulcer bleeding or perforation is extremely low. It also assumes that early diagnosis in the rare patient with malignant disease and no alarm symptoms has little effect on outcome.

However, this strategy has several major limitations. It takes little account of the fact that many dyspeptic people consult their doctor only after months, if not years, of symptoms and self medication. It also fails to meet the expectations of patients who are increasingly informed and often expect referral for investigation or prescription of more powerful drugs. It offers little reassurance to those patients who believe that their symptoms are due to more serious disease. In controlled trials empiric treatment results in the lowest scores for patient satisfaction.

Investigate all patients by early endoscopy
It has been argued that, as most dyspeptic patients end up having some investigation anyway, earlier investigation may prove more cost effective. However, cost effectiveness modelling has shown that if the incidence of peptic ulcer disease in dyspeptic patients is less than 10%, it would take more than five years for the costs of investigation to be recouped in savings from fewer prescriptions. Results of several large trials based in primary care of the cost effectiveness of this approach are expected soon.

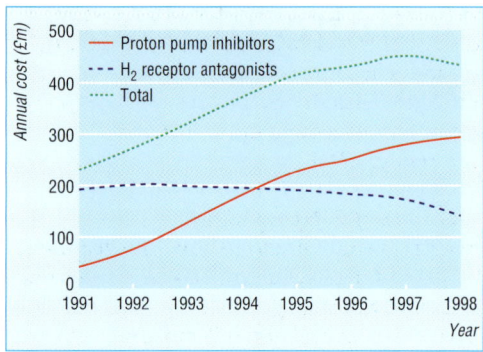

Figure 1.3 Cost of prescriptions for ulcer healing drugs in England and Wales

---

Box 1.2 Why do patients consult with dyspepsia?

Major factors
- Patient's perception of the problem
- Patient's peers' perception of the problem
- Availability of medical care
- Availability of non-medical treatments
- Cost to the patient

Minor factors
- Interference with work, personal life, or physical functioning
- Medicalisation of symptoms

Box 1.3 Causes of dyspepsia

Findings from endoscopy in 2659 patients aged >40 years consulting their doctor for dyspepsia for the first time:

Hiatus hernia or oesophagitis	19%
Peptic ulcer:	
Gastric	6%
Duodenal	10%
Duodenitis	4%
Gastric or oesophageal cancer	3%
Normal (including gastritis only)	59%

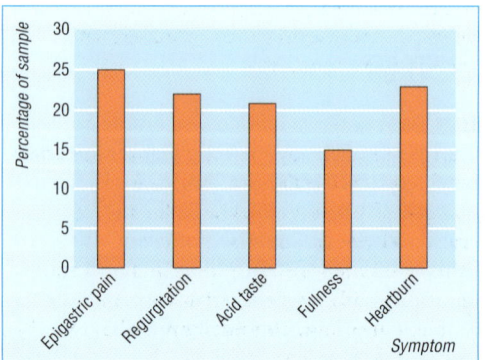

Figure 1.4 Symptoms of dyspepsia reported by UK adults over the previous year

A recent Cochrane review has shown that initial endoscopy may be associated with a 15% relative reduction in symptoms compared with empiric acid suppression. A primary care trial in patients aged over 50 years has shown that this small reduction in symptoms might be cost effective if the unit cost of endoscopy could be kept to £100.

Only investigate a proportion of dyspeptic patients
The rationale behind this proposal is to increase the diagnostic yield of endoscopy without missing any serious causes in those not investigated. Criteria involving age (related to gastric cancer risk), consumption of non-steroidal anti-inflammatory drugs, and "alarm" symptoms have been proposed.

More recently, non-invasive tests for *Helicobacter pylori* have been suggested: lack of *H pylori* infection is a good predictor of the absence of peptic ulcer or gastric cancer. A retrospective study examined the effect of screening for *H pylori* by serology before endoscopy in patients aged under 45 and not taking non-steroidal anti-inflammatory drugs. It found that positive serology was highly predictive of endoscopic abnormalities, and endoscopy workload would have been reduced by 23% if only the patients seropositive for *H pylori* had been investigated. However, recent prospective trials have suggested that in general practices near patient serology tests may lack sufficient accuracy and that the strategy might even increase endoscopic workload.

Test for H pylori and treat
Up to 15% (and higher in some areas such as Glasgow) of dyspeptic patients infected with *H pylori* may have peptic ulcer disease, so there is an argument for treating such patients, without first proving the presence of an ulcer by endoscopy. This may have the added advantage of preventing peptic ulcers or gastric cancer that might develop in the future as well as treating current disease.

However, the successful eradication of *H pylori* requires combination therapy and carries a risk of increasing bacterial resistance. As the prevalence of *H pylori* infection in the developed world is steadily declining, treating patients without testing for infection is unlikely to be cost effective.

In contrast, decision analysis models suggest that testing for *H pylori* and treating those who test positive ("test and treat") is likely to be one of the most cost effective approaches in primary care. Three randomised controlled trials have shown that testing for and treating *H pylori* was as effective as endoscopy based management in controlling symptoms in patients referred to secondary care, but cost less because many fewer endoscopies were performed. However, the long term effects of eradicating *H pylori* in patients without peptic ulcer disease are uncertain, and the effects on resource use compared with empiric acid suppression are unknown.

Role of hospitals
The appropriate management of dyspeptic patients in primary care relies on a combination of making a diagnosis to determine the most effective treatment and reducing the uncertainty experienced by both doctors and patients. In terms of potentially effective treatment two groups of patients should be actively sought— those with peptic ulcer disease, induced either by *H pylori* infection or non-steroidal anti-inflammatory drugs, and those with early gastric cancer.

Endoscopy is not the only investigation that may be used to support management: tests for *H pylori* infection, particularly the highly accurate ^{13}C-urea breath tests and stool antigen tests, may be increasingly important in primary care. Specialists have an important role in coordinating local endoscopy services and in treating patients with difficult to manage dyspepsia.

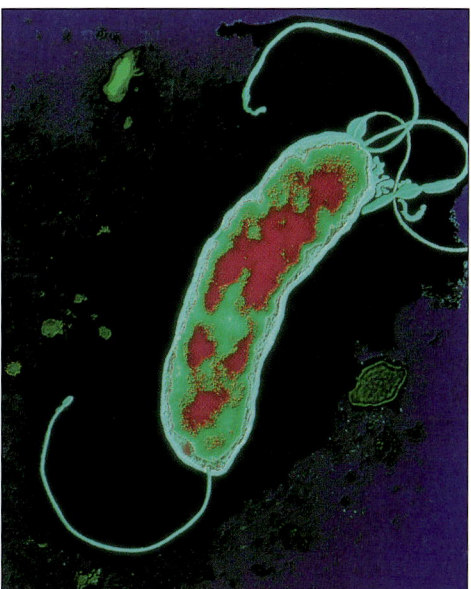

Figure 1.5 Transmission electron micrograph of *Helicobacter pylori*

Clinical summary
- Patients aged under 55 presenting with dyspepsia for the first time should be managed initially with a short course of antacid or antisecretory drugs (based on consensus guidelines)
- Patients still symptomatic should be tested for *H pylori* infection (by laboratory serum enzyme linked immunosorbent assay (ELISA), stool antigen test, or ^{13}C-urea breath test) and, if positive, investigated by endoscopy or given eradication treatment
- Treatment for *H pylori* infection without testing is not recommended as most patients treated will not be infected (cohort study)
- Patients with gastric and duodenal ulceration, newly diagnosed or still requiring treatment, should receive *H pylori* eradication treatment (meta-analysis of randomised trials)
- Unless a major complication has occurred (such as bleeding), cure should be taken as relief of symptoms without proceeding to a breath test (prospective cohort study)
- Patients with persistent symptoms should have a ^{13}C-urea breath test to confirm *H pylori* eradication (consensus guidelines)
- Treatment of asymptomatic *H pylori* infection is not recommended

Indigestion is reproduced with permission of the Wellcome Library. The table of patients consulting with upper gastrointestinal disorders is derived from the Office of National Statistics *Morbidity Statistics from General Practice–Fourth national study 1991-92*. The graph of costs of drug prescriptions is based on data from the Prescription Pricing Authority. The table of causes of dyspepsia is adapted from Hallisey et al, *BMJ* 1990;301:513-5. The graph of prevalence of symptoms of dyspepsia is adapted from Penston and Pounder, *Aliment Pharmacol Ther* 1996;10:83-9. The electron micrograph of *H pylori* is reproduced with permission of Dr Linda Stannard and Science Photo Library.

2 Oesophagus: Heartburn

John de Caestecker

Gastro-oesophageal reflux disease (GORD) is defined as symptoms or mucosal damage (oesophagitis) resulting from the exposure of the distal oesophagus to refluxed gastric contents. However, the symptoms of reflux oesophagitis do not equate with mucosal damage, and patients with endoscopic evidence of oesophagitis do not necessarily have the worst symptoms.

In primary care GORD is therefore best thought of in terms of symptoms: symptom control is the aim of most management strategies, and indeed typical symptoms can guide doctors to the correct diagnosis. Since frequency and intensity of symptoms are poorly predictive of the severity of mucosal damage, with the converse also applying, endoscopy may be less useful than commonly perceived. A variety of other tests are available to diagnose and assess the severity of disease if symptoms are atypical and results of endoscopy normal.

Nevertheless, oesophagitis resulting from GORD has become the commonest single diagnosis resulting from endoscopy carried out for dyspepsia, although whether this represents a true increase in prevalence or simply reflects a change in referral practice is unclear. There is little doubt that a spectrum of severity of disease exists, with most affected people never consulting a doctor and only a minority with unremitting symptoms or complications from the disease receiving attention from hospital specialists. Consequently, treatment of patients presenting in general practice may not be best guided by the outcome of most clinical trials, which have recruited patients from those referred to hospital.

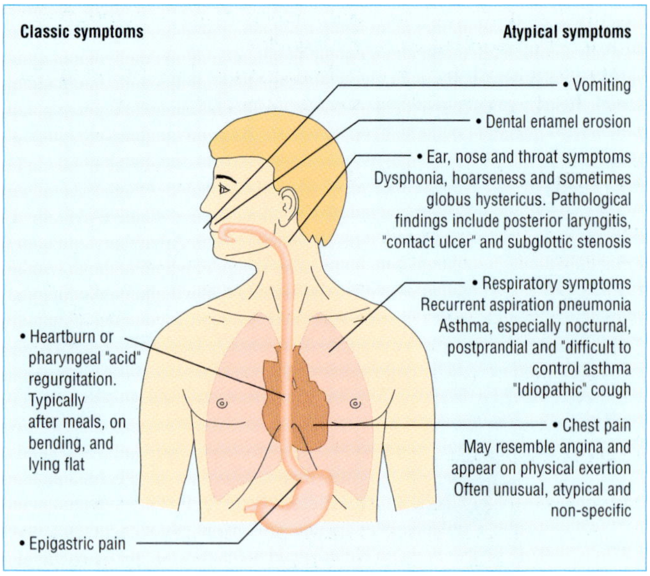

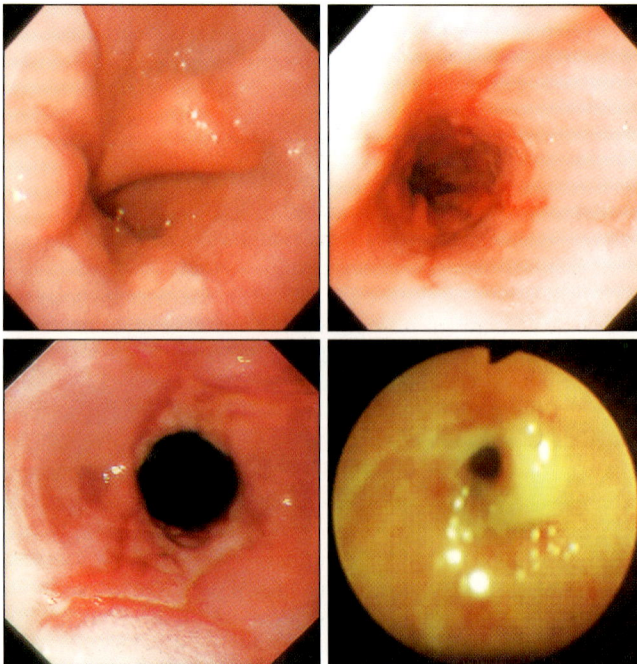

Figure 2.1 Presentation of gastro-oesophageal reflux disease

Terminology and aetiology

Oesophagitis refers to endoscopic or histological evidence of an acute inflammatory process in the oesophagus. Only about 60% of patients in whom GORD is eventually diagnosed have endoscopic evidence of oesophagitis. Some evidence suggests that among patients in the community or those with atypical presenting symptoms the proportion with oesophagitis may be even lower.

Hiatus hernia is present when gastric mucosal folds are observed more than 2-3 cm above the diaphragm by endoscopy or barium radiology and is found in about 30% of people aged over 50 years. However, most patients with an hiatus hernia do not have GORD, but about 90% of patients with marked oesophagitis have hiatus hernia. Thus, hiatus hernia may not result in GORD but can contribute to the disease. Hiatus hernia itself rarely gives rise to symptoms, although a large hernia may undergo torsion (volvulus) to cause acute epigastric or retrosternal pain with vomiting.

Both oesophageal and gastric factors affect the occurrence of reflux. The critical factor is lower oesophageal sphincter incompetence: most reflux occurs during transient relaxation of the lower oesophageal sphincter resulting from failed swallows (swallows not followed by a normal oesophageal peristaltic wave) and gastric distension (mostly after meals). Recent evidence has indicated that the diaphragmatic crural fibres surrounding the oesophageal hiatus act as an external sphincter in concert with the intrinsic lower oesophageal sphincter. Failure of this crural mechanism may allow a hiatus hernia to occur. The hernial sac may additionally provide a sump of gastric contents available for reflux once the lower oesophageal sphincter relaxes. Oesophageal acid clearance depends both on

Figure 2.2 Four grades of endoscopic oesophagitis. Top left: Grade 1 (single erosion with a sentinel fold of gastric mucosa). Top right: Grade 2. Bottom left: Grade 3. Bottom right: Grade 4 (stricture)

swallowed saliva and intact lower oesophageal peristalsis, which is impaired in about 30% of patients with GORD. Gastric acid production is usually normal in GORD, while delayed gastric emptying occurs in about 40%.

Duodenogastro-oesophageal reflux of bile may play a subsidiary role to that of gastric acid and pepsin in patients with an intact stomach and has been implicated in the pathogenesis of Barrett's oesophagus and its sequelae.

Odynophagia, pain on swallowing, should be distinguished from dysphagia, difficulty in swallowing (see next article).

Clinical features and presentation

There is a spectrum of clinical presentation, ranging from symptoms alone to complications resulting from mucosal damage. Up to 40% of patients seen in hospital in whom reflux is eventually diagnosed have symptoms other than classic heartburn or pharyngeal acid regurgitation, including a variety of respiratory and pharyngeal symptoms.

Natural course of GORD

The condition is characteristically chronic and relapsing: in follow up studies at least two thirds of patients continue to take drugs continuously or intermittently for reflux symptoms for up to 10 years. Symptoms disappear in less than a fifth of those taking no drugs, and in the short term endoscopic evidence of oesophagitis may come and go independently of symptoms. There is no evidence that patients inevitably go on to develop severe erosive oesophagitis, Barrett's oesophagus, or stricture.

Symptomatic relapse after discontinuing treatment is common and is chiefly dependent on initial severity of oesophagitis. In studies with large proportions of patients having initial severe oesophagitis, relapse rates of up to 80% at six months have been reported.

Investigation

GORD is a disease of different facets. No single investigation is capable of infallibly diagnosing the condition nor of assuring its relevance to symptoms in an individual case.

Choice of clinical investigation depends on presentation, the patient's age, presence or absence of "alarm" symptoms (such as dysphagia or weight loss), and the question to be answered. Thus, if the question is to decide if mucosal injury is present, endoscopy or barium radiology is most appropriate, whereas an acid perfusion test or 24 hour oesophageal pH monitoring with observation of symptom-reflux association is the most useful test in deciding if symptoms are due to oesophageal acid exposure.

Despite these considerations, in practice endoscopy is the most commonly performed initial investigation, combining inspection of the oesophagus with that of the stomach and duodenum to exclude other causes of dyspepsia. In up to two thirds of patients, however, the results of endoscopy are normal, particularly if patients are taking proton pump inhibitors or H_2 antagonists at the time of investigation.

Therefore, in young patients with longstanding typical symptoms (heartburn or pharyngeal acid regurgitation after meals and with postural changes) no investigation is necessary. Atypical symptoms, dysphagia, or presentation with short duration of symptoms in patients aged over 55 years usually require investigation. There are no a priori grounds for diagnosis or treatment of *Helicobacter pylori* infection in most patients, since there is no evidence at present of an association.

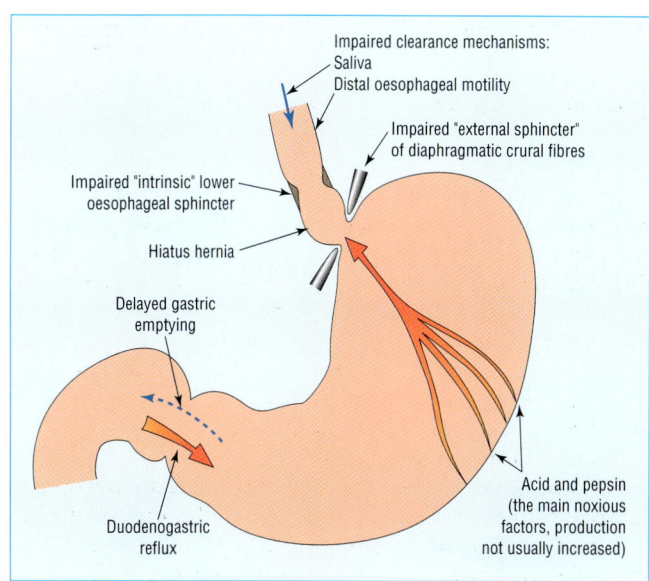

Figure 2.3 Main pathophysiological mechanisms in gastro-oesophageal reflux disease

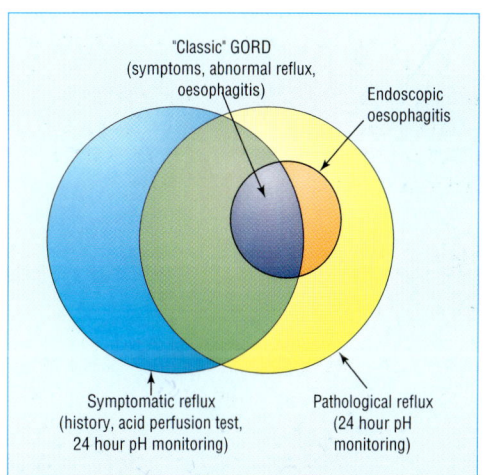

Figure 2.4 Overlap between symptoms, endoscopic evidence of damage, and physiological findings in reflux oesophagitis

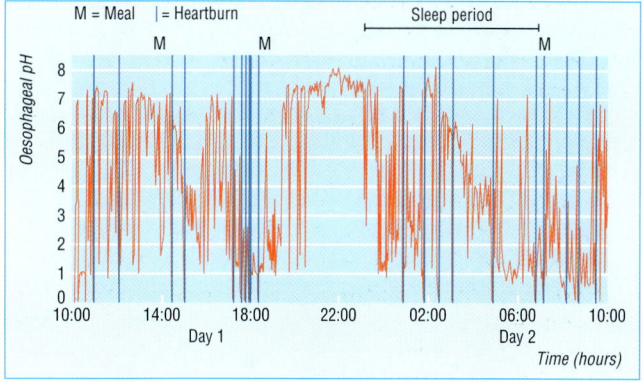

Figure 2.5 24 Hour recording of oesophageal pH in patient with gastro-oesophageal reflux disease but normal endoscopic appearance. Note close association between symptoms and reflux and large amount of daytime and night time reflux. (Reflux = intraoesophageal pH ≤ 4)

Indeed, there is some evidence that eradication of infection, if present, may actually make acid suppression with proton pump inhibitors more difficult in GORD.

Treatment

Aims
For most patients, the aim is acceptable symptom control using the least treatment necessary to achieve this. Therefore, if symptom control is the aim, endoscopy to assess healing of oesophagitis is unnecessary. Indeed, it is now known that, at least for patients treated with proton pump inhibitors, absence of symptoms on treatment equates with healing of oesophagitis.

For those with complications, such as stricture or bleeding from oesophagitis, the aim will be long term healing of oesophagitis.

Patients with Barrett's oesophagus have a risk of between 1 in 50 and 1 in 200 of developing adenocarcinoma of the oesophagus. Many gastroenterologists therefore recommend yearly or biennial endoscopic screening with multiple biopsies to detect dysplasia. Patients with severe dysplasia often have an undetected early cancer and so are offered oesophagectomy. Surveillance of patients with Barrett's oesophagus to detect severe dysplasia or early cancer is controversial, partly because its benefits have not been established by well designed randomised controlled trials. Clearly a surveillance policy is inappropriate in elderly patients who are unfit for surgery. Endoscopic ablation of the abnormal columnar mucosa in Barrett's oesophagus by photodynamic laser or thermal methods looks promising and may become standard treatment. It must be combined with high doses of proton pump inhibitors or antireflux surgery to prevent continuing acid reflux.

General measures
Patients should be advised to lose weight if overweight. There is no formal evidence to support this assertion, but success (though rarely achieved) may result in improved symptom control. Raising the head of the bed on 15 cm wooden blocks has been shown in a controlled trial to improve symptoms and healing of oesophagitis. There is little evidence that avoidance of specific foods has much effect on the course of the disease, but many patients have already identified and stopped eating foods that produce symptoms before consulting their doctor. Other potentially damaging drug treatment should also be reviewed.

While the benefits associated with these general measures may be unproved, they allow patients to be involved with decision making and may help them avoid over-medicalising their condition.

Antacids and alginates
Antacids are effective for short term relief of symptoms. Although their efficacy is difficult to confirm in controlled trials, many sufferers, particularly those who do not consult a doctor, rely on self medication with antacids. Alginates work by forming a floating viscous raft on top of the gastric contents that provides a physical barrier to prevent reflux. To maximise this effect, they are therefore best taken after meals, otherwise they rapidly empty from the stomach and thus give only transient relief of symptoms by virtue of their antacid content.

Acid suppression therapy
The two major classes of agent available are the H_2 receptor antagonists and the proton pump inhibitors. There is little doubt that proton pump inhibitors are more rapidly and

---

Box 2.1 Investigations for gastro-oesophageal reflux disease

Barium radiology
Strengths
- Good for structural lesions (such as stricture) and detection of motor abnormalities

Weaknesses
- Poor for assessing minor mucosal abnormalities
- Detection of "free" reflux of barium is insensitive (40%) though specific (90%) for GORD

Endoscopy
Strengths
- Best for assessment of oesophagitis
- May detect other potential causes of symptoms
- Allows for biopsy

Weaknesses
- Detection of oesophagitis is insensitive for GORD (<60%)

24 hour oesophageal pH monitoring
Strengths
- Patients monitored at home, where symptoms are most likely to occur
- Can quantify reflux and measure association with symptoms
- Useful for atypical presentations if other tests are normal and to confirm adequate acid suppression if poor response to treatment
- New probes can detect bile reflux

Weaknesses
- Expertise required for interpretation, so not available in all centres
- Time consuming
- Normal result does not exclude GORD

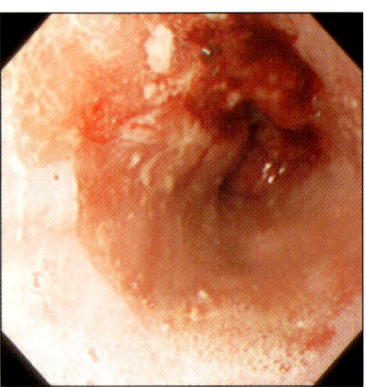

Figure 2.6 Endoscopic view of cancer in a Barrett's oesophagus

---

Box 2.2 General measures for managing gastro-oesophageal reflux disease

- Assess use of drugs—Avoid non-steroidal anti-inflammatory drugs (associated with benign strictures) and if possible avoid or reduce dose of nitrates, calcium channel antagonists, and anticholinergics
- Avoid or reduce smoking—However, this may be counterproductive as it often results in weight gain
- Avoid large evening meals and food or drink within 3 hours of bed time—Have smaller meals spread through day
- Avoid or reduce fats or chocolate
- Avoid or reduce any food or drink that is causing a problem—Problems have been found with citrus fruits, fruit juices, tea and coffee, peppermint, onions, garlic, cinnamon, cloves

---

Box 2.3 Complications of reflux oesophagitis

- Often present without preceding or other symptoms of reflux, especially in elderly patients
- Haematemesis or melaena
- Iron deficiency anaemia
- Dysphagia due to benign stricture, or cancer in Barrett's oesophagus

completely effective for both relieving symptoms and healing oesophagitis, regardless of disease severity. Because of this, a cost effectiveness argument has been made in favour of proton pump inhibitors as first choice treatments in all cases. However, the data on which these calculations have been made have generally come from hospital based clinical trials and may not be applicable to general practice.

Many patients in primary care may achieve good and lasting symptom relief from short intermittent courses of H_2 receptor antagonists at standard doses (such as ranitidine 150 mg twice daily or cimetidine 400 mg twice daily). For patients with severe or refractory oesophagitis, particularly those with complications such as stricture, proton pump inhibitors are the drugs of choice. The optimal daily dose for most patients is omeprazole 20 mg, lansoprazole 30 mg, pantoprazole 40 mg, or rabeprazole 20 mg, but higher doses may give additional clinical benefit in patients with resistant oesophagitis. For most patients, there is no clinical advantage in choosing one proton pump inhibitor over another.

Motility modifying drugs
These include metoclopramide and domperidone. Although both relieve symptoms of heartburn to a degree similar to H_2 receptor antagonists, they do not heal oesophagitis. In addition, metoclopramide has a relatively high incidence of side effects on the central nervous system. However, these drugs may be useful, particularly in patients with other dyspeptic symptoms such as nausea or early satiety.

Maintenance treatment
Only proton pump inhibitors, at standard or half standard doses, have been shown to be effective agents for maintenance of remission in those who require it. Indications for maintenance treatment include
- Severe oesophagitis, especially presenting with complications (such as stricture, bleeding, peptic ulcers)
- Barrett's oesophagus (although there is no evidence that continuous treatment prevents evolution to cancer)
- Symptoms (typical or atypical) relapsing as soon as treatment is stopped.

Surgery
Laparoscopic anti-reflux surgery seems to be as successful as conventional surgery in controlling reflux in the short term without the disadvantages of a long hospital stay or convalescence. It has become an increasingly popular option for patients requiring long term medical treatment. The results from a randomised controlled trial comparing surgery with maintenance drug treatment are awaited.

Further reading
- National Institute of Clinical Excellence. *Guidance on the use of proton pump inhibitors in the treatment of dyspepsia.* London: NICE, 2000
- Dent J, Brun J, Fendrick AM, Fennerty MB, Janssens J, Kahrilas PJ, et al. An evidence-based appraisal of reflux disease management—the Genval workshop report. *Gut* 1999;44(suppl 2):S1-16
- Lundell L, ed. *Guidelines for the management of symptomatic gastro-oesophageal reflux disease.* London: Science Press, 1998

Box 2.4 Factors to consider when choosing a proton pump inhibitor
- Efficacy of drugs similar at equivalent doses, but lansoprazole 30 mg may be equivalent to omeprazole 40 mg daily
- Pantoprazole and lansoprazole have the highest bioavailability and thus most predictable effects
- Clinically important drug interactions are rare
- Pantoprazole has least induction of cytochrome P450 and thus least potential for interaction with metabolism of other drugs (such as warfarin, theopyllines, benzodiazepines, phenytoin)
- Side effects rare and minor with all proton pump inhibitors

---

Box 2.5 Treatment strategy for gastro-oesophageal reflux disease

Mild GORD
(No or mild oesophagitis, symptoms mild or moderate)
"Step up" strategy
- Start with general measures (antacids and alginates)
- If ineffective try H_2 receptor antagonist at standard dose for 4-6 weeks
- Reserve proton pump inhibitors for those with poor symptom relief
- Suitable for many patients in general practice
- Endoscopic monitoring unnecessary
- "Step down" strategy an alternative—Start with proton pump inhibitors and reduce to minimal effective treatment

Severe GORD
(Severe oesophagitis possibly with bleeding, strictures, or peptic ulcers within a Barrett's oesophagus)
"Step down" strategy
- Start with proton pump inhibitors for 8 weeks
- Reduce to maintenance treatment with half dose if possible
- If patient presented with bleeding or peptic ulcer endoscopic confirmation of healing is needed. May require high dose of proton pump inhibitor (such as omeprazole 40 mg daily)

Atypical symptoms
(Such as respiratory symptoms, ear, nose, and throat symptoms)
- Prolonged treatment with proton pump inhibitors, often at high dose (such as omeprazole 40 mg daily)
- Confirmation of GORD desirable by pH monitoring
- Confirm adequate acid suppression by pH monitoring if no response

---

Box 2.6 Indications for surgical treatment
- Poor response to medical treatment
  Failure to suppress acid reflux should be confirmed
- Persisting "volume reflux"
  Regurgitation of gastric contents without heartburn on maximal medical treatment
  Occurs especially at night
  Risk of aspiration
- Difficult benign strictures requiring frequent dilation despite medical treatment
- Patient's choice among those requiring long term maintenance treatment, including younger patients with Barrett's oesophagus

3 Oesophagus: Atypical chest pain and motility disorders

John Bennett

Chest pain has been a diagnostic problem for centuries. Heberden's superb clinical description of angina pectoris (and other chest pains) still stands, but today's doctors may be no better at diagnosing cardiac pain accurately than their predecessors 60 years ago. Even when a doctor is sure that the pain is non-cardiac, the more inquiring patient often wants a more specific label.

Much of the interest in this subject has arisen from the extensive investigation of patients concerned that their symptoms could be cardiac in origin. Given the associated and inevitable selection bias, there is little objective evidence on which to base practice, but the oesophagus is undoubtedly one of the organs that can generate problematic chest pain.

This article describes the oesophageal disorders responsible, and ways to diagnose them. Psychological factors are often important in patients with chest pain, so that common sense, understanding a patient and his or her problem, and good communication are usually more important than diagnostic tests and powerful drugs.

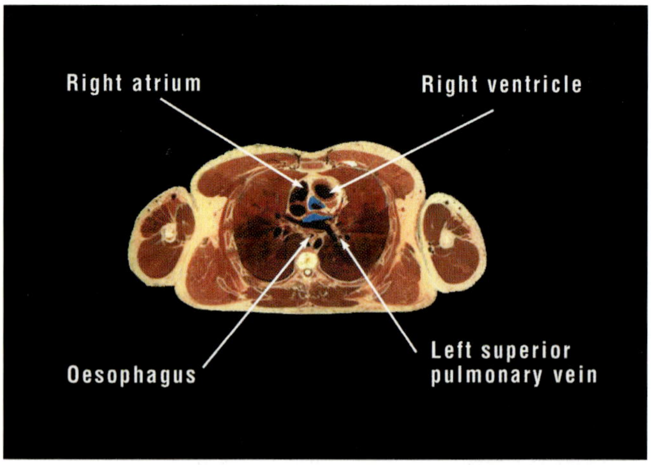

What does oesophageal pain feel like?

Oesophageal pain has many patterns: it is often described as burning, sometimes as gripping, and it can also be pressing, boring, or stabbing. Usually in the anterior chest, it tends to be felt mainly in the throat or epigastrium and sometimes radiates to the neck, back, or upper arms—all of which may equally apply to cardiac pain. The commonest patterns of cardiac and oesophageal pains are quite different and well recognised, but perhaps 20% of each are much harder to feel confident about.

Mechanisms of oesophageal pain

Discomfort or pain from the oesophagus may arise from irritant stimuli to the mucosa or from mechanical effects on the muscular wall, each with different sets of receptors.

Mucosal stimulation
Atypical chest pain arising from oesophageal mucosal irritation can be imitated by infusing hydrochloric acid into the oesophagus. This causes discomfort in most people eventually, but, for it to be truly acid induced, it must resolve rapidly when perfusion ceases (Bernstein test).

When the level of exposure of the lower oesophagus to acid is measured by a pH probe, two things can be seen. Firstly, atypical chest pain is usually associated with a drop in pH, but many episodes of acid reflux are painless. Secondly, there may be little relation between the amount of acid reflux and the severity and frequency of atypical chest pain. This parallels the longstanding observation that some patients with marked oesophagitis have little or no heartburn.

Other factors must therefore be involved in the threshold for experiencing pain, and these are discussed below.

Mechanical changes
Distension of the oesophagus, by swallowing a large food bolus or experimentally by inflating a balloon in its lumen, will cause pain in most people. However, individuals with recurrent

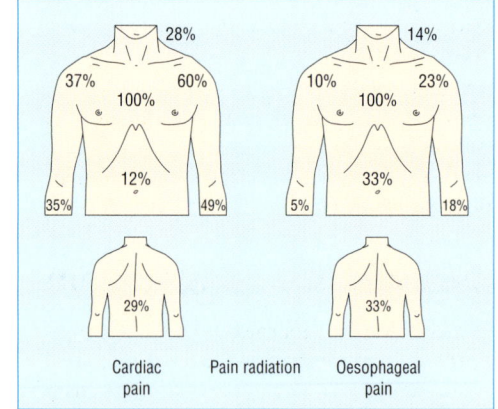

Figure 3.1 The close proximity of the heart and oesophagus mean that distinguishing oesophageal from cardiac pain is often difficult

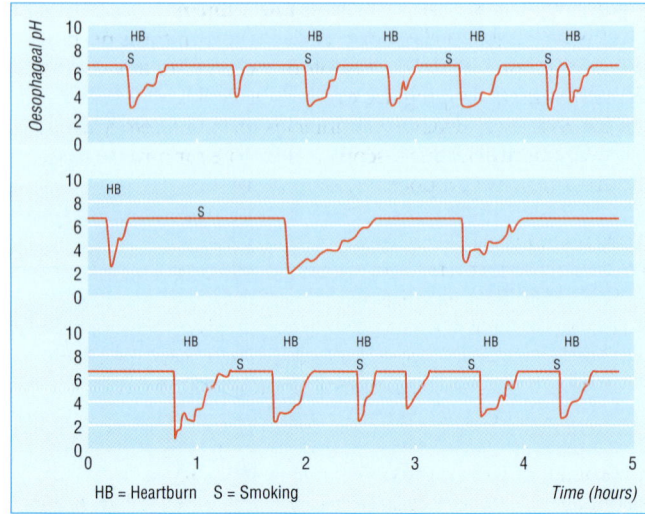

Figure 3.2 Frequency of pain experienced in different anatomical sites by patients with cardiac pain and oesophageal pain

Figure 3.3 Intraoesophageal pH tracing showing frequent episodes of acid reflux, some of them associated with heartburn

spontaneous chest pain experience pain at much lower inflation volumes, suggesting that they have a "lowered threshold." Others may have induced distension because they have a high threshold for belching.

Altered motility of the oesophagus (sometimes loosely referred to as "spasm") can be a cause of chest pain. The rare condition of diffuse oesophageal spasm (seen radiologically as a "corkscrew oesophagus") is associated with pain, and so is achalasia. Powerful, prolonged contractions can be induced by injection of edrophonium and may cause simultaneous pain, but similar contractions may also be seen in patients without chest pain. When pressures in the oesophagus are monitored continuously for 24 hours, a few patients with recurrent chest pain can be seen to have pain episodes associated with various abnormalities of oesophageal contractions, but this is surprisingly uncommon.

Pain threshold—psychological factors

Patients with other sorts of painful syndromes, such as irritable bowel syndrome or fibromyalgia, also feel pain induced by balloon distension of the oesophagus more readily than people without pain syndromes.

These observations led to the concept of "altered visceral receptor sensitivity." When such individuals are given standard psychological tests many are found to have greater anxiety, depression, somatisation, neuroticism, or even panic disorder scores than control subjects, and some studies have shown improvement in pain with the use of antidepressants or anxiolytics.

Moreover, some abnormalities of oesophageal motility—including "non-specific motility disorder" and "nutcracker oesophagus"—can be induced by the unconscious gulping and hyperventilation performed by some anxious individuals. Unfortunately, well intentioned but misguided medical interventions aimed at excluding cardiac disease may worsen this by raising patients' anxiety and medical dependency.

Managing possible oesophageal pain

This can be a difficult problem, complicated by the fact that both oesophageal problems and ischaemic heart disease are relatively common in middle age and can coexist. Diagnosis of one does not exclude the other. However, first ensure that the patient is not taking sumatriptan for migraine; this drug causes chest pain in 3-5% of those taking it.

Atypical chest pain associated with heartburn

Patients with atypical chest pain and reflux symptoms need no investigation provided their symptoms respond to advice on diet and weight, stopping use of non-steroidal anti-inflammatory drugs, or to antacids or antisecretory drugs (see previous article). Endoscopy is desirable for anyone with alarm symptoms or a poor response to treatment.

"Pain like angina"

If the pain has elements that suggest a cardiac origin—such as an association with exercise, radiation to neck, jaw, or arms, or the presence of cardiac risk factors (family history, smoking, hypertension, obesity, hypercholesterolaemia, etc)—then the heart must first be investigated with resting and exercise electrocardiograms. If these are normal then the often difficult choice must be made between more invasive cardiac tests (such as coronary angiography, thallium scanning, etc) or oesophageal tests; specialist referral may be indicated, with the choice between cardiologist or gastroenterologist determined by the nature of the pain.

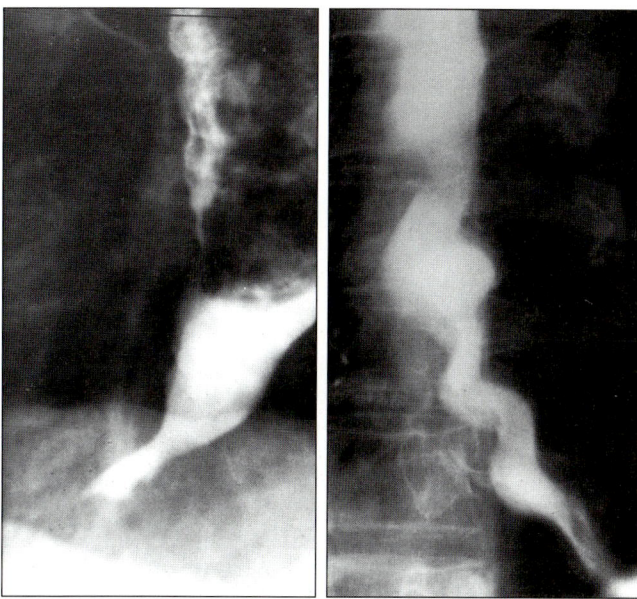

Figure 3.4 Barium swallow radiographs showing achalasia (left) and diffuse oesophageal spasm ("corkscrew oesophagus") (right)

Box 3.1 Primary oesophageal motility disorders

Achalasia
- Absent distal peristalsis
- Abnormal relaxation of lower oesophageal sphincter

Diffuse oesophageal spasm
- Simultaneous contractions
- Intermittent peristalsis

Hypertensive ("nutcracker") oesophagus
- Increased contraction amplitude (mean > 180 mm Hg)
- Normal peristalsis

Ineffective oesophageal motility
- Contractions of low amplitude or failed and non-transmitted

---

> Sumatriptan causes chest pain in up to 5% of migraineurs

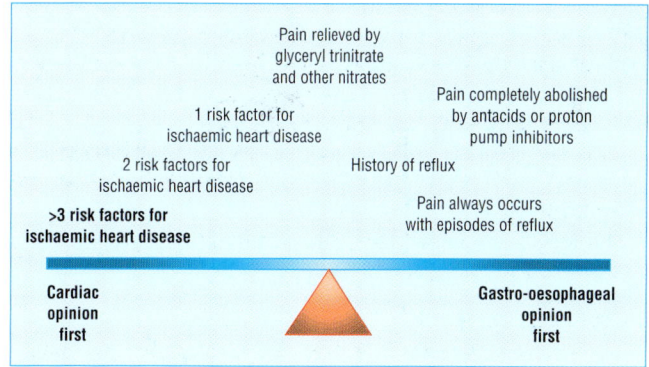

Figure 3.5 Choices for proceeding with patients with chest pain and normal electrocardiograms

ABC of the Upper Gastrointestinal Tract

All tests create anxiety in patients and their family, and can lead to medical dependence. This is especially so when tests are "on the heart." Studies show that, even when oesophageal tests are positive, patients and their family doctors often continue to believe that their pain originates from the heart.

Before referring any patient to a specialist, a general practitioner should have a clear idea of what may be achieved and explain the risks and benefits to the patient. A period of sympathetic and supportive observation may often be the best initial approach. This will not always be successful, and some patients can absorb substantial health resources in visits to doctors, use of drugs, and urgent "false alarm" admissions to coronary care units. Resident junior doctors wishing to consider an oesophageal cause for atypical chest pain should adopt the following approach.

Investigating the oesophagus as a cause of atypical chest pain
Some patterns of symptoms make it likely that chest pain is oesophageal in origin: an association with meals, dysphagia, relief by antacids, associated acid reflux, and a history of heartburn.

If reflux is suggested then an empiric approach may be appropriate. For patients with severe pain or dysphagia, endoscopy is the usual initial investigation (to look for oesophagitis, cancer, or other gastric disease), but a barium swallow (recorded on video by an experienced radiologist well briefed about the symptoms) will give more information about motility problems such as diffuse spasm or achalasia.

A "therapeutic trial" with high dose proton pump inhibitors (double healing doses) is an alternative approach with the attraction of simplicity, and if the pain disappears promptly and completely it is highly likely that reflux is the cause of the pain. However, it is important to remember that a misleading "placebo response" is common, particularly in anxious patients, and it is always an error to continue such drugs if the symptomatic response is only partial.

If endoscopy or barium swallow fail to confirm the diagnosis 24 hour pH monitoring is necessary to detect any abnormal acid reflux as the most likely treatable cause of "spasm." If there is no abnormal reflux, and the pain continues as a significant problem, further tests are available to detect an oesophageal origin, although the treatment is far from effective.

Oesophageal manometry
  Stationary—This may show subtle motility abnormalities not revealed by radiology, but all too often it shows only "non-specific" motility disorders, which are often clinically irrelevant.
  Ambulatory—This is relatively simple for patients but involves complex technology in obtaining the records and analysing them. It can, however, be useful in patients with intractable problems, revealing abnormalities such as intermittent spasm and their association with episodes of pain, especially in patients with intermittent dysphagia.

Oesophageal provocation tests
  Pharmacological—Edrophonium can be injected during stationary oesophageal manometry to provoke abnormal contractions and pain that patients can compare with their spontaneous symptoms. However, abnormal contractions can occur in normal individuals, and patients may anticipate symptoms.
  Chemical—Acid perfusion of the oesophagus can similarly reveal recognisable pain.
  Mechanical—Balloon distension may show both an increased sensitivity to pain and that the pain is indeed oesophageal.

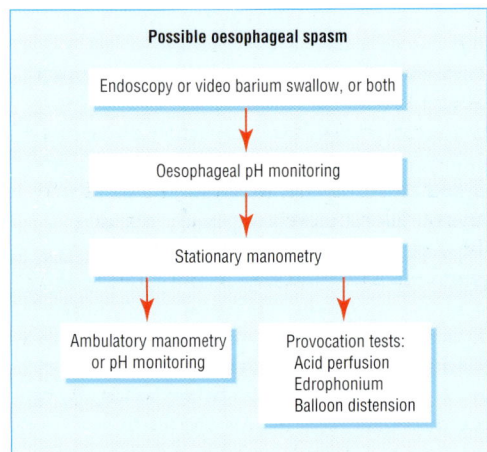

Figure 3.6 Progression of tests for investigating the oesophagus as a cause of chest pain

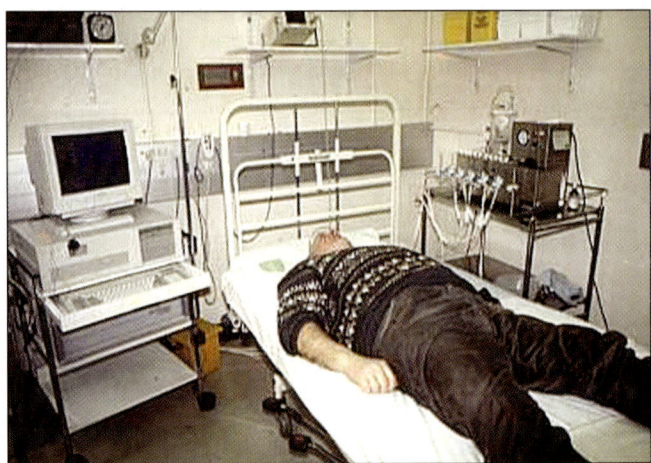

Figure 3.7 Stationary oesophageal manometry is an outpatient procedure taking about 30 minutes to perform. A polyvinyl tube about 4 mm in diameter is passed pernasally after topical anaesthesia. The tube consists of several microcapillary tubes connected to external pressure transducers, which pass signals to a computer for real time display. Measurements of distal oesophageal pressure are taken during swallows of water while the tube is slowly withdrawn from the stomach

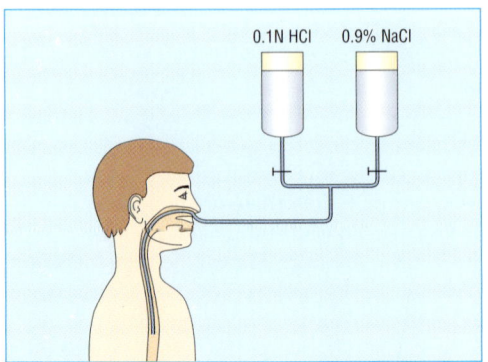

Figure 3.8 The acid perfusion test for chemical provocation of the oesophagus

Treatment

The most important aspect of treating oesophageal pain is a sympathetic appraisal of patients' problems. Are they mainly worried about their heart or does their pain interfere with life in some other way, or is their family most concerned?

Any reflux element is readily treated by the range of safe antisecretory drugs of different levels of power; "titrating upwards" is the best way to use them. If response seems inexplicably inadequate, pH monitoring while taking the drug can help.

Psychological problems need considerate management with both drugs and psychotherapy as appropriate. Tricyclic antidepressants (such as amitriptyline 25-75 mg at night) may be particularly useful because of their known value in functional somatic pain disorders such as irritable bowel syndrome.

When a true spasm disorder is demonstrated by manometry, physical treatment may have a place. Achalasia (and sometimes diffuse spasm) may be helped by judicious balloon dilatation of the gastro-oesophageal sphincter, but this carries the risk of perforation or subsequent gastro-oesophageal reflux. There are reports (all uncontrolled) of use of long oesophagomyotomy, but this is an invasive approach for a relatively benign disorder.

Nitrates and calcium channel blocking drugs can be tried—taken sublingually for episodes of pain or orally and regularly as a prophylactic. Separating useful effects from placebo ones is not easy, and these drugs have not been proved in randomised clinical trials. They have two disadvantages, however. One is that patients, reassured they do not have angina, may have their confidence undermined when they read the datasheet and realise they are taking antianginal drugs. The other is that any latent reflux may be accentuated.

Anticholinergic drugs (the traditional "antispasmodics") have no useful effect, and it is illogical to prescribe metoclopramide or other prokinetic agents.

Box 3.2 Treatments for oesophageal spasm

Reflux
- Antisecretory drugs

Anxiety or depression
- Explanation and reassurance
- Psychotherapy
- Anxiolytics
- Tricyclic antidepressants

Achalasia
- Balloon dilatation
- Cardiomyotomy
- Botulinum toxin

Other spasm disorders
- Nitrites
- Calcium channel blockers
- Possibly balloon dilatation

The cross sectional view of a human torso is adapted from the Visible Human Project. The list of primary oesophageal motility disorders is adapted from Richter JE. *Lancet* 2001;358:823-8.

4 Dysphagia

William Owen

Dysphagia is a distressing symptom and indicates a delay in the passage of solids or liquids from the mouth to the stomach. It is sometimes difficult to understand why patients may take so long to consult their doctor for advice, but whenever patients present a diagnosis should be urgently sought. Dysphagia should be distinguished from odynophagia, which is discomfort or pain on swallowing hot or cold liquids and, occasionally, alcohol.

In clinical practice it is useful to separate those causes that predominantly affect the pharynx and proximal oesophagus (high dysphagia) and those mostly affecting the oesophageal body and oesophagogastric junction (low dysphagia).

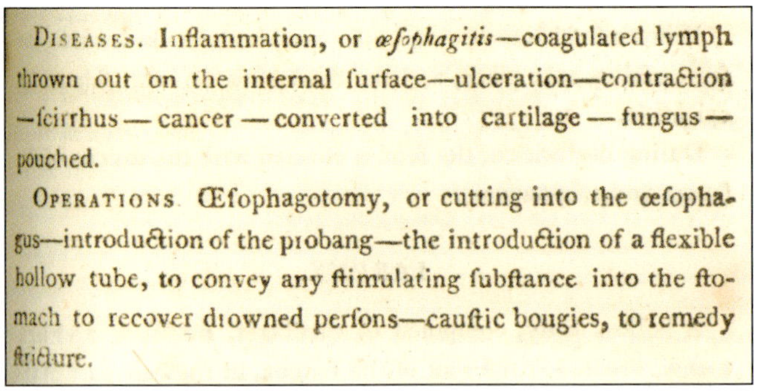

Management of high dysphagia

There may be pointers in a patient's history to a neuromuscular cause of high dysphagia such as neurological disease or a tendency for spillage into the trachea when the patient eats, producing coughing or choking. A patient may find it easier to swallow solids or semisolids rather than liquids and may also complain of nasal regurgitation of food. High dysphagia must be differentiated from globus hystericus (the feeling of having a lump in the throat without any true dysphagia). Globus is a common symptom, and when the patient is examined no abnormality is usually found. It is believed to be a functional disorder but is sometimes associated with gastro-oesophageal reflux.

Generally, radiology is often more rewarding than endoscopy in clarifying the cause of high dysphagia. Cineradiography with liquid barium and bread soaked in barium may give valuable functional as well as anatomical information about the pharynx and cricopharyngeal segment. Most problems are related to failure of pharyngeal contraction or to cricopharyngeal relaxation, or a combination of both.

For patients with a pouch or a cricopharyngeal bar, surgical myotomy of the overactive cricopharyngeus with, if appropriate, pouch excision is the treatment of choice in most cases.

Other causes of upper dysphagia are more difficult to manage. In patients recovering from a stroke who need feeding, a fine bore, soft feeding tube can be passed down under radiological guidance. Passage of a large soft oesophageal bougie under light sedation can occasionally alleviate the symptoms, but if the problem is chronic and disabling then a percutaneous endoscopic gastrostomy—in which a gastrostomy tube is passed into the stomach via a percutaneous abdominal route under the guidance of an endoscopist—can be considered.

Management of low dysphagia

The main concern with low dysphagia is that a patient may be harbouring a malignancy. The patient's history may give clues to this, such as a short duration of symptoms (less than four months), a progressive differential dysphagia affecting solids more than liquids, or considerable weight loss. If, however, the problem has existed for several years, equal difficulty is experienced with solids and liquids, and there is no weight loss, then achalasia is a more likely cause.

A patient's history may be misleading, however. Localisation of the point of dysphagia can be poor and patients with an obstructing carcinoma of the cardia occasionally localise the point of obstruction to the throat. Patients with a reflux stricture

Figure 4.1 The use of bougies to remedy dysphagia caused by oesophageal stricture has been a standard treatment for centuries. (Reproduced from Robert Hooper's *The Anatomist's Vade-Mecum* 1805)

Box 4.1 Causes of high dysphagia affecting pharynx and cricopharyngeus

Neurological
- Stroke
- Parkinson's disease
- Cranial nerve palsy or bulbar palsy (such as multiple sclerosis, motor neurone disease)

Anatomical or muscular
- Myasthenia gravis
- Oropharyngeal malignancy (uncommon)
- Cricopharyngeal spasm
- Pharyngeal pouch

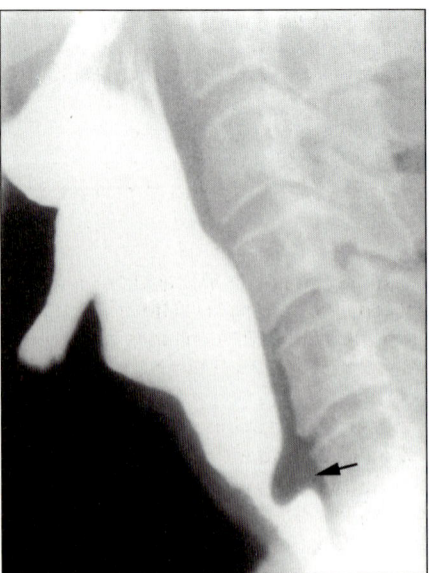

Figure 4.2 Barium swallow showing cricopharyngeal spasm (arrow)

Box 4.2 Causes of low (oesophageal) dysphagia
- Carcinoma of oesophagus or oesophagogastric junction (cardia)
- Reflux disease with or without stricture
- Motility disturbance of oesophagus (such as achalasia, scleroderma, or diffuse oesophageal spasm)

may have no history suggestive of gastro-oesophageal reflux (the so called silent refluxers), and Barrett's oesophagus is often characterised by diminished oesophageal sensitivity and lack of pain. Patients with achalasia may complain of chest pain and minor dysphagia only, and the condition may sometimes mimic gastro-oesophageal reflux.

Endoscopy is usually the best way to determine the cause of dysphagia because of its high diagnostic accuracy and the opportunity to take biopsies or to proceed to dilatation, if appropriate, at the same time.

Procedure after endoscopy

Endoscopy will usually reveal a benign peptic stricture, an obvious tumour, or no abnormality.

Management of peptic stricture

Peptic stricture is usually due to gastro-oesophageal reflux, but drugs such as non-steroidal anti-inflammatory drugs, potassium supplements, or alendronic acid are occasional causes. The differential diagnosis also includes caustic strictures after ingestion of corrosive chemicals, fungal strictures, and postoperative strictures.

The diagnosis should be confirmed by biopsy or cytology, and the stricture then dilated. Often only one dilatation is needed, but re-dilatation over the next few months may be needed. Proton pump inhibitors reduce the rate of re-stricturing, and thus the need for re-dilatation, and are therefore recommended long term.

Occasionally, a patient with a seemingly benign stricture fails to respond to dilatation, and the dysphagia rapidly recurs even after repeated procedures. In such cases malignancy should be suspected, and this may become obvious only after repeat biopsy or brush cytology.

The risk of rupture after oesophageal dilatation is about 0.5%. Should a perforation occur the patient is managed conservatively with a strict "Nil by mouth" regimen, intravenous antibiotics, nasogastric drainage, and proton pump inhibitors. A follow up radiological examination a few days later nearly always shows satisfactory healing of the perforation. If the patient becomes severely shocked after rupture, however, surgery may be needed to treat this life threatening condition.

Barrett's oesophagus
Barrett's oesophagus (columnar lined oesophagus) arises as a result of a longstanding acid (and bile) reflux. The oesophageal epithelium undergoes metaplasia so that it changes from the usual pale squamous epithelium to a pink columnar epithelium that resembles gastric mucosa.

The risk of developing an adenocarcinoma of the oesophagus is increased about 80-fold with this condition, and cancer is heralded by the development of high grade dysplasia in the oesophagus. In the absence of high grade dysplasia or frank carcinoma the finding of Barrett's oesophagus does not pose an enormous risk to the patient. Controversy still exists as to whether regular surveillance is justified because the risk of developing oesophageal carcinoma is about 1 per 50-200 years of patient follow up. The risk of developing carcinoma is greater if there is a long segment (>7 cm) of Barrett's oesophagus.

Provided there is no significant dysplasia it is appropriate to reassure the patient and manage conservatively in the usual way, probably with endoscopic surveillance every one to two years. There is no evidence that long term treatment with a proton pump inhibitor or antireflux surgery either causes regression of Barrett's oesophagus or abolishes the risk of developing cancer. Barrett's oesophagus may also cause

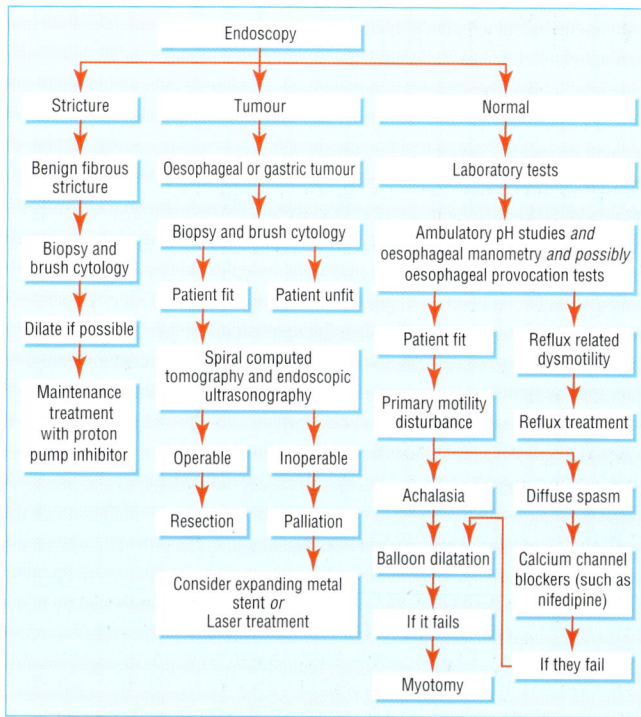

Figure 4.3 Algorithm for endoscopic management of dysphagia

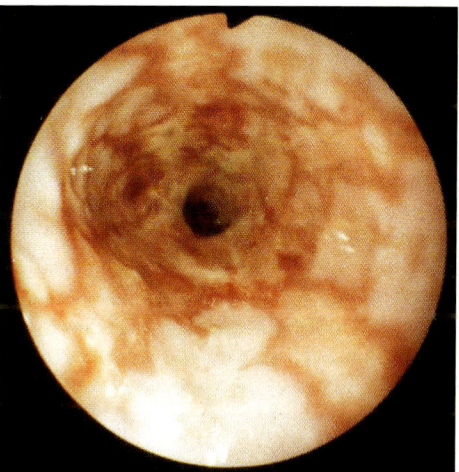

Figure 4.4 Endoscopic appearance of benign oesophageal stricture with associated severe reflux

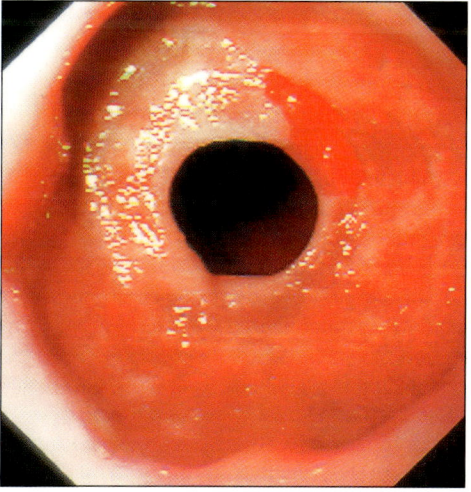

Figure 4.5 Endoscopic appearance of Schatzki's ring (constriction of the lower oesophagus)

ABC of the Upper Gastrointestinal Tract

dysphagia because of an associated benign stricture, which usually responds to simple dilatation and medical management.

Management of a tumour

If endoscopy reveals a tumour a decision has to be made whether treatment is potentially curative or merely palliative.

Potentially curative treatment

The diagnosis should be confirmed by biopsy or brush cytology. It is essential that the patient should undergo rigorous staging before a resection is considered. An upper age limit of 75 years seems sensible, although fitness is clearly important and rules are made only for guidance. Major cardiovascular or respiratory problems militate against operating. Spiral computed tomography and endoscopic ultrasonography (if available) give valuable information about the size of the primary tumour as well as the presence of any metastases. Palliative resection is usually contraindicated if a liver metastasis is present because of the poor results and high mortality.

The operation usually entails an oesophagogastrectomy, as most tumours now are near the oesophagogastric junction. The hospital mortality in specialised tertiary centres well versed in the technique is in the order of 5%, but the five year survival is still only about 25%. Several centres have reported that use of preoperative adjuvant chemotherapy gives a modest improvement in survival at three years. The current trend is that all cases of adenocarcinoma of the lower oesophagus that have breached the oesophageal wall (T3 and T4) are to be given downstaging chemotherapy for three or six cycles and then be reassessed to determine the operative status. The expectation is that this will result in an improved long-term survival although definite data on this are not yet available.

Digestive function after an oesophagectomy is surprisingly good, and patients should return to a normal diet within a few weeks of leaving hospital. Patients may occasionally develop dysphagia due to an anastomotic stricture; this is amenable to endoscopic dilatation, but tumour recurrence must be excluded.

If the biopsy shows a squamous cell tumour, which is usually found in the middle or upper oesophagus, external beam radiotherapy may be a good alternative to surgery in older patients. Intraluminal radiotherapy (brachytherapy) is an attractive alternative and a faster mode of treatment.

Palliative treatment

A tumour may be considered unresectable because of doubts about a patient's general fitness, because computed tomography or endoscopic ultrasonography shows that it involves adjacent vital structures such as the aorta or trachea, or because metastases are present.

The restoration of swallowing is the prime objective in such patients, and the recent development of self expanding metal stents, which can expand up to 20 mm in diameter, has radically changed clinical practice. The stents are a great advance over the old tubes and can be inserted either endoscopically or radiologically. Possible complications include stent migration and growth of the tumour through the mesh. However, stent design is evolving rapidly, such as partly covered stents to prevent ingrowth of tumour and improved shape to minimise migration. Bleeding and perforation are rare complications.

Laser recanalisation of oesophageal cancer also offers an effective way of improving patients' ability to swallow. This may have to be repeated at regular intervals, but it is particularly suitable for high tumours, where stents are uncomfortable, and for protuberant growths at the oesophagogastric junction. Alcohol injection into the tumour in an attempt to shrink it is used in some centres.

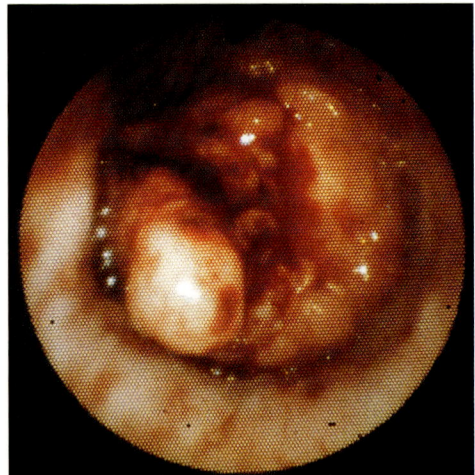

Figure 4.6 Endoscopic appearance of carcinoma of the oesophagus

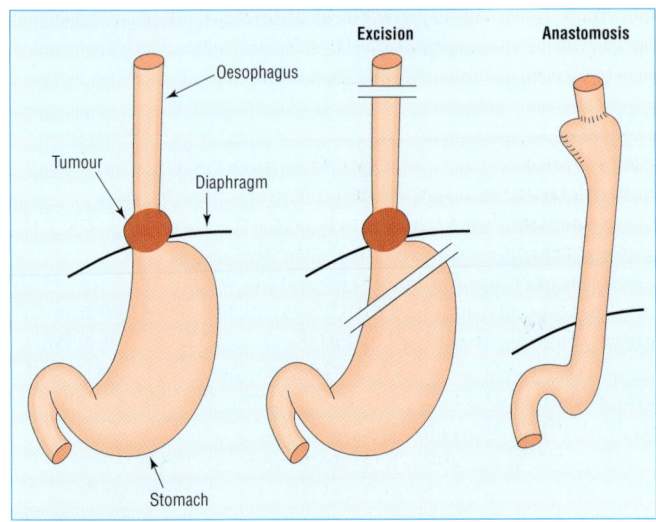

Figure 4.7 Oesophagogastrectomy of an oesophageal tumour, involving excision of the distal part of the oesophagus and the proximal stomach followed by anastomosis

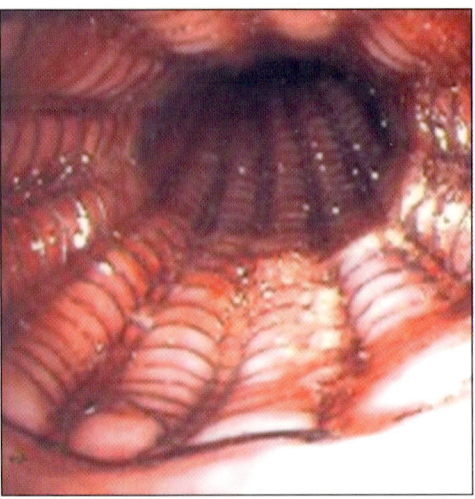

Figure 4.8 Endoscopic view of an inserted oesophageal stent

Box 4.3 Problems associated with oesophageal stents

- Migration
- Perforation
- Tumour overgrowth
- Obstruction
- Pain
- Bleeding
- Reflux or aspiration

Dysphagia with normal endoscopic appearance
If endoscopy shows no obvious abnormality a diagnosis of a primary motility disturbance of the oesophagus such as achalasia should be considered.

Achalasia
Achalasia may be missed at endoscopy, and radiology is positive in only about 70% of cases. Oesophageal manometry will confirm the diagnosis of achalasia by showing the absence of oesophageal peristalsis and a non-relaxing lower oesophageal sphincter.

Pneumatic balloon dilatation of the lower oesophageal sphincter will often relieve the dysphagia, and if dilatations are repeated (up to three) the success rate can be up to 77%. Patients should be warned about the risk of rupture of the oesophagus (<5%), which can be detected on a post-dilatation radiological study. If the patient fails to respond to balloon dilatation, then a Heller's myotomy of the lower oesophageal sphincter is recommended by either laparoscopic or open technique. This will improve the swallowing in most patients although there is a small risk (10-15%) of inducing postoperative gastro-oesophageal reflux.

Other causes of dysphagia
Laboratory investigations may reveal other causes of dysphagia in the presence of a normal endoscopy.

Reflux related dysmotility—These patients should be managed with the standard treatment for acid reflux.

Diffuse oesophageal spasm—This is a uncommon disorder of oesophageal motility characterised by repetitive non-peristaltic waves affecting the body of the stomach (see previous article).

Monilial (candidal) oesophagitis can be a rare complication of treatment with antibiotics or inhaled corticosteroids or may occur in immunosuppressed patients.

AIDS related oesophagitis can be caused by cytomegalovirus, herpesvirus, or fungal disease.

Conclusion

In patients presenting with dysphagia, the cause is usually an obstruction. The differential diagnosis lies between oesophagogastric malignancy, reflux disease with a stricture, or a motility disturbance. The duration of the problem is probably the most valuable clinical guide to the diagnosis, and endoscopy is the most rewarding investigation.

The image of an inserted stent is reproduced with permission of Jeremy Livingstone.

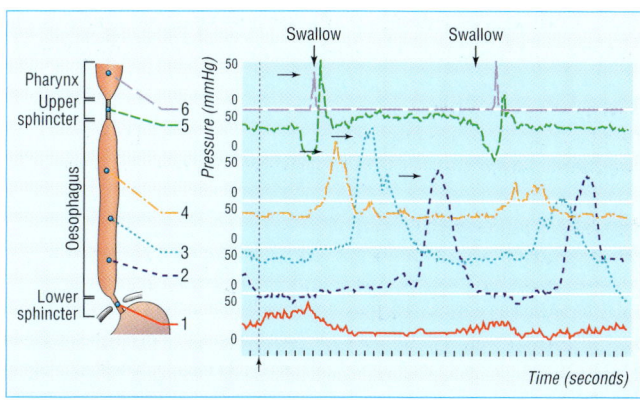

Figure 4.9 Normal recording at oesophageal manometry (horizontal arrows indicate progression of normal oesophageal peristalsis)

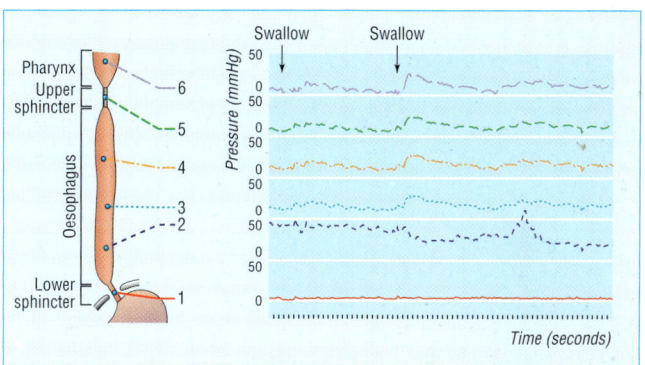

Figure 4.10 Oesophageal manometry in achalasia of the cardia, showing lack of peristalsis and a non-relaxing lower oesophageal sphincter

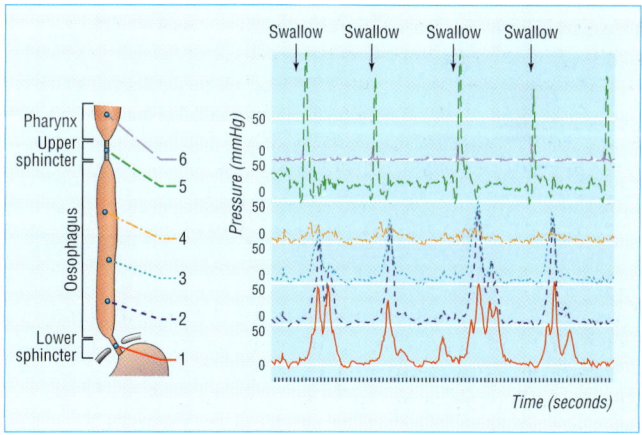

Figure 4.11 Oesophageal manometry in diffuse oesophageal spasm, showing synchronous multipeaked high pressure waves

5 Epidemiology and diagnosis of *Helicobacter pylori* infection

Robert P H Logan, Marjorie M Walker

Helicobacter pylori is a small, curved, highly motile, Gram negative bacillus that colonises only the mucus layer of the human stomach. Since its discovery in 1984, it has been recognised as the principal cause of peptic ulcer disease and as the main risk factor for the development of gastric cancer. However, most infected people (>70%) are asymptomatic. We therefore need to discover how infection is acquired, why ulcers or cancer occur in so few of those infected, and how this subgroup can be identified and treated.

Epidemiology of *H pylori* infection

H pylori is one of the commonest bacterial pathogens in humans. The prevalence of infection varies but is falling in most developed countries. Seropositivity increases with age and low socioeconomic status. Retrospective seroepidemiological studies have shown a cohort effect consistent with the hypothesis that infection is mainly acquired in early childhood. Until recently, however, it has been difficult to assess accurately the incidence (or route) of infection because of the inaccuracy and cost of detecting (non-invasively) *H pylori* in young children. Primary acquisition in adults, or reinfection after successful eradication, does occur but is less common, with an annual incidence of 0.3-0.7% in developed countries and 6-14% in developing countries.

How *H pylori* is usually acquired and its route of transmission are unknown. Since humans are the only known reservoir of infection, it is likely that in developed countries *H pylori* is picked up from siblings, other children, or parents, predominantly via the gastro-oral route. In developing countries faecal-oral transmission may also occur. Various risk factors are associated with *H pylori* infection, but the extent to which these are simply markers of childhood socioeconomic deprivation is unclear. *H pylori* infection is an occupational hazard for gastroenterologists and is associated with performing endoscopy.

Why is *H pylori* a chronic infection?

Although *H pylori* initially induces an acute inflammatory gastritis, this immunological response by the host is generally not sufficient to clear infection, which persists for life. In addition, infection with one strain of *H pylori* does not protect against subsequent co-infection with a different strain. Infection with multiple strains is quite common and occurs more frequently in developing countries. Polyclonal infection allows DNA to be exchanged between different strains, which could promote the spread of genes encoding important virulence factors or resistance to antibiotics.

H pylori is not a new bacteria species and, by virtue of its urease enzyme and other products, has become extremely well adapted to its unique niche within the gastric mucus. It also has considerable genetic heterogeneity (no two strains are identical), and studies have suggested that this diversity may allow each strain to become uniquely adapted to each host to an extent that, for some subjects, it may be considered as a commensal bacteria.

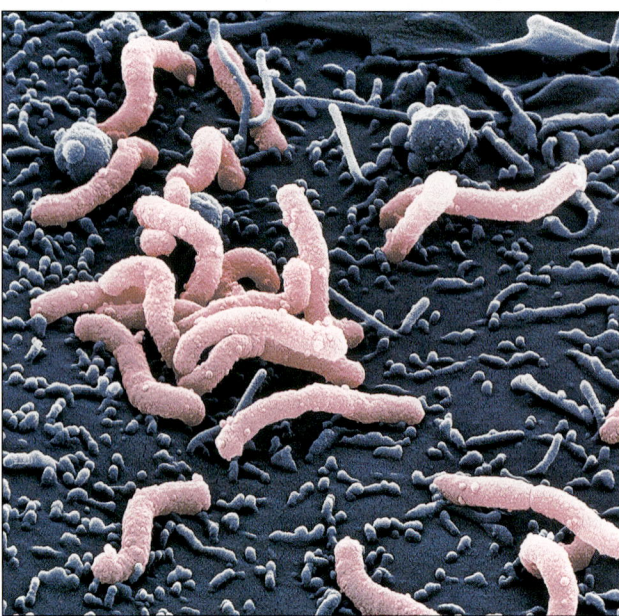

Figure 5.1 Coloured scanning electron micrograph of *H pylori* on surface of gastric cell

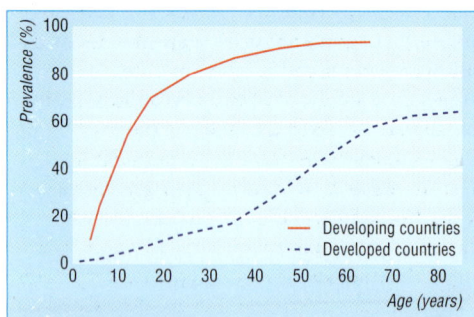

Figure 5.2 Prevalence of *H pylori* infection by age in developing and developed countries

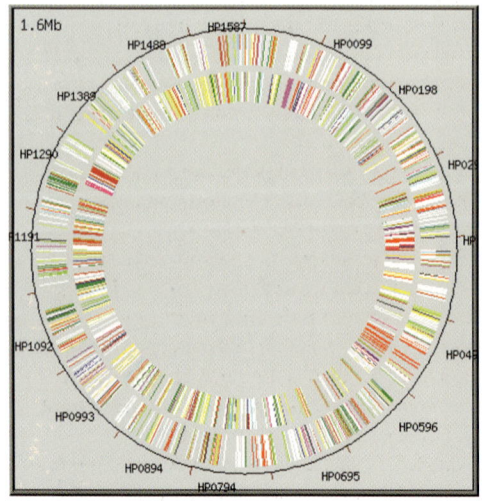

Figure 5.3 Circular display of the *H pylori* genome. The recent sequencing of the whole genome of two separate *H pylori* strains will help in developing new treatments and emphasises the importance of *H pylori* as a human pathogen

Peptic ulcer and gastric cancer

About 15% of infected individuals will develop peptic ulcer (duodenal or gastric) or gastric cancer as a long term consequence of infection. The outcome of infection depends mainly on the severity and topography of histological gastritis, which may be determined by the age at which infection is acquired. Infection in infancy is thought to lead to pangastritis, whereas acquisition in later childhood may lead to a predominantly antral gastritis only.

With antral gastritis there is loss of regulatory feedback (but with an intact and undamaged acid secreting gastric corpus), and the high acid load reaching the duodenum leads to the development of duodenal gastric metaplasia. The islands of gastric metaplasia are subsequently colonised by *H pylori*, leading to duodenitis and a high risk of duodenal ulcer.

In contrast, pangastritis, with an inflamed corpus, is associated with the loss of acid secreting cells, which leads to an increased risk of gastric ulcer and gastric cancer—similar to that seen with autoimmune gastritis in pernicious anaemia.

Diagnosis

Invasive tests

H pylori can be detected at endoscopy by histology, culture, or urease tests, each with inherent advantages and disadvantages. All these biopsy based methods for detecting *H pylori* are liable to sampling error because infection is patchy. Up to 14% of infected patients do not have antral infection but have *H pylori* elsewhere in the stomach, especially if they have gastric atrophy, intestinal metaplasia, or bile reflux. In addition, after partially effective eradication treatment, low levels of infection can easily be missed by endoscopic biopsy, leading to overestimates of the efficacy of eradication treatment and reinfection rates. Proton pump inhibitors affect the pattern of *H pylori* colonisation of the stomach and compromise the accuracy of antral biopsy. Consensus guidelines therefore recommend that multiple biopsies are taken from the antrum and corpus for histology and for one other method (either culture or urease testing).

Histology—Although *H pylori* may be recognised on sections stained with haematoxylin and eosin alone, supplementary stains (such as Giemsa, Genta, Gimenez, Warthin-Starry silver, Creosyl violet) are needed to detect low levels of infection and to show the characteristic morphology of *H pylori*. An important advantage of histology is that, in addition to the historical record provided, sections from biopsies (or even additional sections) can be examined at any time, and that gastritis, atrophy, or intestinal metaplasia can also be assessed. Biopsy specimens from other parts of the stomach can be retained in formalin to be processed only if antral histology is inconclusive.

Culture—Microbiological isolation is the theoretical gold standard for identifying any bacterial infection, but culture of *H pylori* can be unreliable. Risks of overgrowth or contamination make it the least sensitive method of detection, and it is the least readily available test for use with endoscopy. Although only a few centres routinely offer microbiological isolation of *H pylori*, the prevalence of multiresistant strains makes it increasing likely that culture and antibiotic sensitivity testing may become a prerequisite for patients with persistent infection after initial or repeated treatment failure.

Urease tests are quick and simple tests for detecting *H pylori* infection but indicate only the presence or absence of infection. The CLO test and cheaper "home made" urease tests are of similar sensitivity and specificity. However, the sensitivity of urease tests is often higher than that of other biopsy based methods because the entire biopsy specimen is placed in the

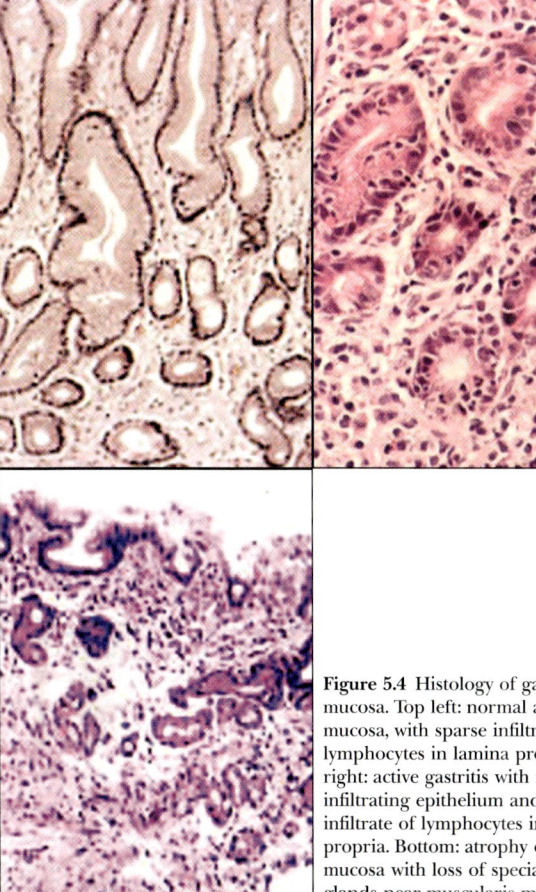

Figure 5.4 Histology of gastric mucosa. Top left: normal antral mucosa, with sparse infiltrate of lymphocytes in lamina propria. Top right: active gastritis with neutrophils infiltrating epithelium and marked infiltrate of lymphocytes in lamina propria. Bottom: atrophy of antral mucosa with loss of specialised glands near muscularis mucosa

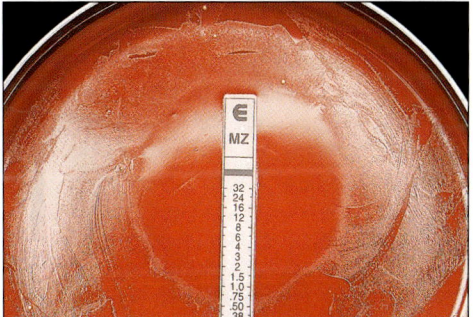

Figure 5.5 Culture of *H pylori* tested for antibiotic sensitivity with an E strip that is impregnated with a scale of increasing concentrations of metronidazole

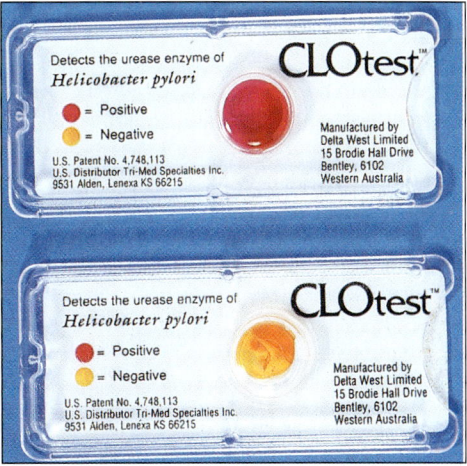

Figure 5.6 Positive and negative results of CLO test for *H pylori*. The urease of *H pylori* hydrolyses urea to release ammonia, which is detected colorimetrically

ABC of the Upper Gastrointestinal Tract

media, thereby avoiding the additional sampling or processing error associated with histology or culture. The sensitivity of biopsy urease tests seems to be much lower (~60%) in patients with upper gastrointestinal bleeding, but this can be improved by placing multiple biopsy samples into the same test vial.

Non-invasive tests

Serology
H pylori infection elicits a local mucosal and a systemic antibody response. Circulating IgG antibodies to *H pylori* can be detected by enzyme linked immunosorbent assay (ELISA) antibody or latex agglutination tests. These tests are generally simple, reproducible, inexpensive, and can be done on stored samples. They have been used widely in epidemiological studies, including retrospective studies to determine the prevalence or incidence of infection.

Individuals vary considerably in their antibody responses to *H pylori* antigens, and no single antigen is recognised by sera from all subjects. The accuracy of serological tests therefore depends on the antigens used in the test, making it essential that *H pylori* ELISA is locally validated. In elderly people with lifelong infection, underlying atrophic gastritis has been associated with false negative results. Consumption of non-steroidal anti-inflammatory drugs has also been reported to affect the accuracy of ELISAs.

Antibody titres fall only slowly after successful eradication, so serology cannot be used to determine *H pylori* eradication or to measure reinfection rates. Although titres of IgM antibodies to *H pylori* fall with age, there are no reliable IgM assays to indicate recent acquisition, which, since this is usually asymptomatic, makes it difficult to identify cases of primary infection and thus establish possible routes of transmission.

An important advantage of serological methods over other tests for *H pylori* infection has been the development of simple finger prick tests that use a fixed, solid phase assay to detect the presence of *H pylori* immunoglobulins. These "near patient tests" (NPT) can be performed in primary care and are much simpler than the ^{13}C-urea breath test, which is the only other test for *H pylori* that is currently used as a NPT. However, the accuracy of the serological NPT is lower than that reported for standard ELISA tests using the same antigen preparations. These tests are often used to reassure patients, but to date no studies have compared the accuracy, cost effectiveness, and reassurance value of the ^{13}C-urea breath test with the serological NPT in primary care.

Urea breath test
Non-invasive detection of *H pylori* by the ^{13}C-urea breath test is based on the principle that a solution of urea labelled with carbon-13 will be rapidly hydrolysed by the urease enzyme of *H pylori*. The resulting CO_2 is absorbed across the gastric mucosa and hence, via the systemic circulation, excreted as $^{13}CO_2$ in the expired breath. The ^{13}C-urea breath test detects current infection and is not radioactive. It can be used as a screening test for *H pylori*, to assess eradication and to detect infection in children. The similar but radioactive ^{14}C-urea breath test cannot be performed in primary care.

Faecal antigen test
In the stool antigen test a simple sandwich ELISA is used to detect the presence of *H pylori* antigens shed in the faeces. Studies have reported sensitivities and specificities similar to those of the ^{13}C-urea breath test (>90%), and the technique has the potential to be developed as a near patient test. The main advantage of the test, however, is in large scale epidemiological studies of acquisition of *H pylori* in children.

Table 5.1 Comparative accuracy, availability, and costs of tests for *H pylori* infection

Test	Sensitivity	Specificity	Availability	Cost
Invasive				
Histology	88-95%	90-95%	+ + + +	££££
Culture	80-90%	95-100%	+ +	£££
Urease test	90-95%	90-95%	+ + + +	£-££
Non-invasive				
^{13}C-UBT	90-95%	90-95%	+ + + +	£££
^{14}C-UBT	86-95%	86-95%	+ + +	££
Serology:				
ELISA	80-95%	80-95%	+ + +	£
NPT	60-90%	70-85%	+ + + +	££
Stool antigen	90-95%	90-95%	+ +	££

UBT = urea breath test. NPT = near patient test.

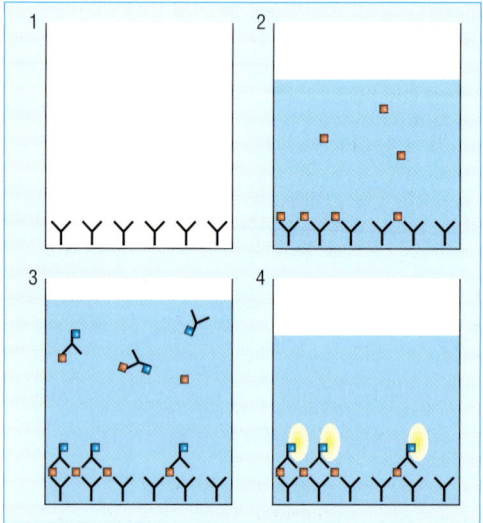

Figure 5.7 Principle of the faecal antigen test. Polyclonal antibody to *H pylori* is adsorbed to microwells (1). Diluted patient samples are added to the wells, and any *H pylori* in the faecal sample is bound to the adsorbed antibody (2). A second *H pylori* antibody conjugated to peroxidase is added and binds to *H pylori* (3). After unbound material is washed off, a substrate is added that reacts with bound peroxidase enzyme to produce a yellow colour (4), the intensity of which can be measured to estimate *H pylori* levels

Further reading
- Graham DY. Helicobacter pylori infection in the pathogenesis of duodenal ulcer disease and gastric cancer: a model. *Gastroenterology* 1997;113:1983-91
- Misiewicz JJ, Harris A. *Clinician's manual on Helicobacter pylori*. London: Science Press, 1995

The electron micrograph of *H pylori* is reproduced with permission of Juergen Berger (Max-Planck Institute) and Science Photo Library.

6 Pathophysiology of duodenal and gastric ulcer and gastric cancer

John Calam, J H Baron

Duodenal and gastric ulcers and gastric cancer are common and serious diseases but occur in only a minority of people infected with *Helicobacter pylori*. Mass eradication of *H pylori* is impractical because of the cost and the danger of generating antibiotic resistance, so we need to know how to target prophylaxis. Knowledge of the mechanisms that lead to ulcer formation or to gastric cancer in the presence of *H pylori* infection is therefore valuable.

Various factors affect the outcome of *H pylori* infection, including the host response and particularly the extent and severity of gastric inflammation and thus the amount of acid secreted by parietal cells. *H pylori* can elevate acid secretion in people who develop duodenal ulcers, decrease acid through gastric atrophy in those who develop gastric ulcers or cancer, and leave acid secretion largely unchanged in those who do not develop these diseases.

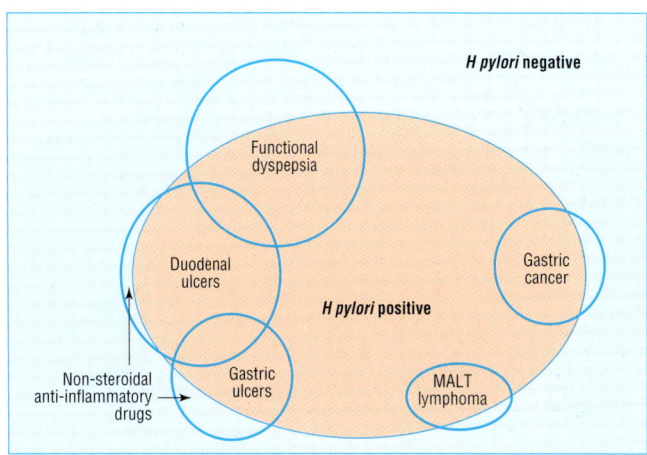

Figure 6.1 Relation of *H pylori* infection to upper gastrointestinal conditions

Regulation of gastric acid secretion

Several specialised cells in the gastric mucosa contribute to the control of acid secretion. G cells in the gastric antrum release the hormone gastrin. Gastrin acts on the enterochromaffin-like cells in the gastric corpus to release histamine, which stimulates parietal cells to secrete acid. Gastrin also stimulates parietal cells directly and promotes growth of enterochromaffin-like and parietal cells.

Histamine H_2 receptor antagonists act by blocking the effect of histamine on parietal cells. Proton pump inhibitors act by inhibiting the enzyme in parietal cells that catalyses acid production for release into the gastric lumen. G cells, enterochromaffin-like cells, and parietal cells are all regulated by release of the inhibitory peptide somatostatin from somatostatin cells, which are distributed throughout the stomach. The effect of *H pylori* infection on acid secretion depends on which part of the stomach is most inflamed because this determines which of these cells are affected most.

H pylori related acid secretion

Hypersecretion in duodenal ulcer disease

Before the discovery of *H pylori* it was known that patients with duodenal ulcers secrete about twice as much acid as controls because they have twice as many parietal cells. Patients with gastric ulcer and those with functional dyspepsia have normal acid output and parietal cell count. Thus there was good evidence that acid played a major role in ulcer formation. Duodenal ulcers did not occur in achlorhydric people or in those secreting < 15 mmol/h of acid. Duodenal ulcers can be healed, but not cured, by pharmacological suppression of acid secretion below this threshold.

Areas of gastric metaplasia in the duodenum can be colonised by *H pylori*, causing inflammation (duodenitis) and leading to further damage of the mucosa. The extent of gastric metaplasia is related to the amount of acid entering the duodenum—lowest in patients with pernicious anaemia who secrete no acid and highest in patients with acid hypersecretion due to gastrin-secreting tumours (Zollinger-Ellison syndrome).

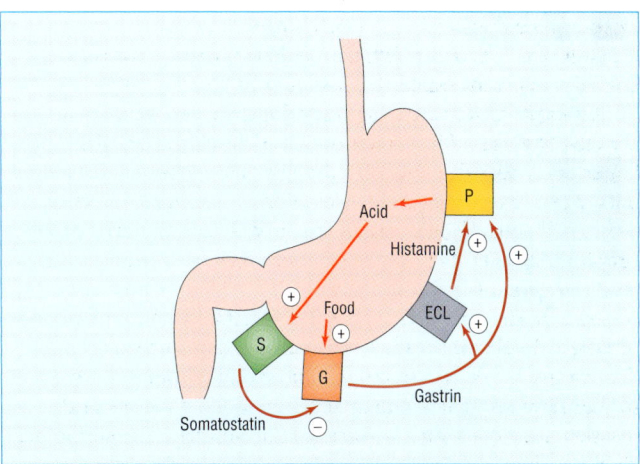

Figure 6.2 Autoregulation of acid secretion. Food stimulates release of gastrin from antral G cells (G). Gastrin stimulates enterochromaffin-like cells (ECL) to release histamine, which stimulates parietal cells (P) in the gastric corpus to secrete acid. Acid stimulates release of somatostatin from somatostatin cells (S) in the antrum, inhibiting further gastrin release

---

Box 6.1 Causes of duodenal ulcer

- *Helicobacter pylori* antral gastritis
- Non-steroidal anti-inflammatory drugs

Rare causes
- Crohn's disease
- Hypergastrinaemia
  Idiopathic
  Gastrinoma
- Hyperparathyroidism

ABC of the Upper Gastrointestinal Tract

Acid hypersecretion in duodenal ulcer disease is virtually always due to *H pylori* infection because secretion returns to normal after the infection is eradicated. The predominantly antral gastritis in duodenal ulcer disease leads to acid hypersecretion by suppressing somatostatin cells and increasing gastrin release from the G cells in the gastric antrum.

Hyposecretion in patients at risk of gastric cancer

H pylori infection predisposes to distal gastric cancer, but patients who develop this complication have diminished acid secretion. Low acid secretion in gastric cancer was, until recently, thought to be predominantly due to gastric corpus gastritis, the associated gastric atrophy leading to loss of parietal cells. However, *H pylori* associated acid hyposecretion can in part be reversed by eradicating *H pylori*, suggesting that hyposecretion is due to inflammation rather than to permanent loss of cells.

H pylori associated acid hyposecretion may also be due to incomplete recovery from the loss of acid secretion that occurs with acute infection or may be in part genetically determined because it is more common in the first degree relatives of patients with gastric cancer.

Low acid secretion predisposes to gastric cancer by several mechanisms, including impaired absorption of vitamin C and overgrowth of salivary and intestinal bacteria within the stomach. By contrast, proximal gastric cancer (at the gastro-oesophageal junction) is associated with normal acid output. The rising incidence of this type of gastric cancer may reflect the decreasing prevalence of *H pylori* infection in Western societies.

Relation between distribution of gastritis and acid secretion

Thus distribution of *H pylori* gastritis determines acid secretion and the clinical outcome of *H pylori* infection, be that duodenal ulcer, gastric ulcer, gastric cancer, or asymptomatic infection. Positive feedback may perpetuate the different patterns of gastritis; for example, suppression of acid with a proton pump inhibitor diminishes antral gastritis but allows *H pylori* to colonise the corpus, which then becomes inflamed. This shows that acid secretion normally protects the corpus from *H pylori* infection. This effect has several important consequences:

- High acid secretion in people with duodenal ulcers may be self perpetuating because it restricts gastritis to the antrum, leaving a healthy corpus to continue secreting acid
- Low acid secretion may be self perpetuating because it increases corpus gastritis, which further depresses acid secretion
- Proton pump inhibitors may be more effective in patients with *H pylori* infection than in those without because they promote corpus gastritis, which further inhibits acid secretion

Aspects of the environment, bacterium, or host that affect acid output or the severity of corpus gastritis might steer a person infected with *H pylori* to a state of high acid secretion (predominantly antral gastritis) or to low acid secretion (predominantly corpus gastritis). This model is attractive because it allows studies of gastric physiology to be integrated with other equally important determinants of disease outcome.

Other factors that might affect gastric physiology and disease outcome

The pathogenic importance of *H pylori* depends on the interaction between bacterial virulence, the host, and the environment.

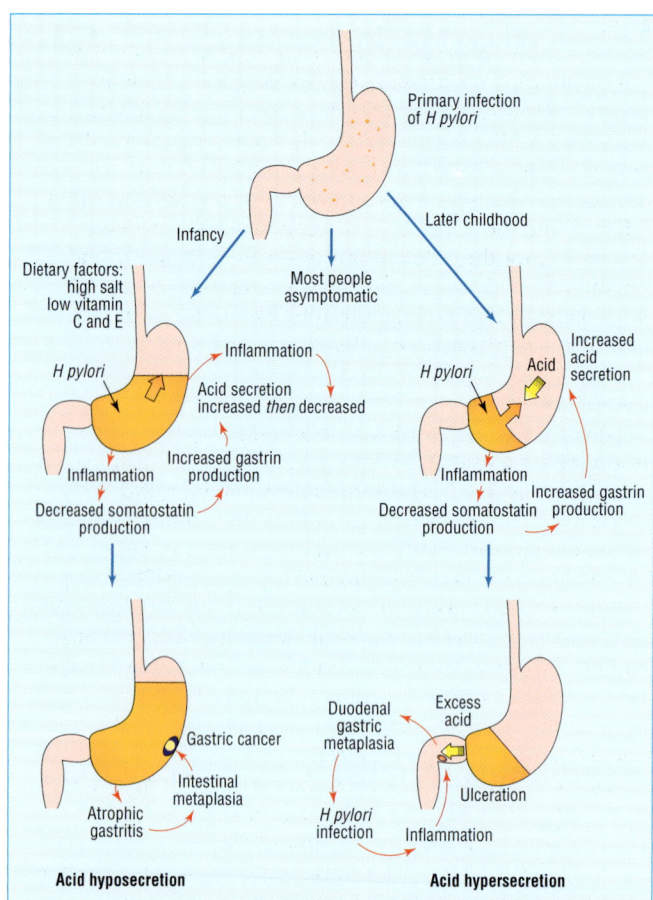

Figure 6.3 With acid hyposecretion (left), the main effect of *H pylori* gastritis affecting the gastric body is to suppress parietal cells, leading to low acid secretion, which is associated with gastric cancer. With acid hypersecretion (right), antral *H pylori* gastritis increases acid secretion by suppressing somatostatin and elevating gastrin release, increasing the risk of duodenal ulceration. Orange areas indicate extent and location of gastritis

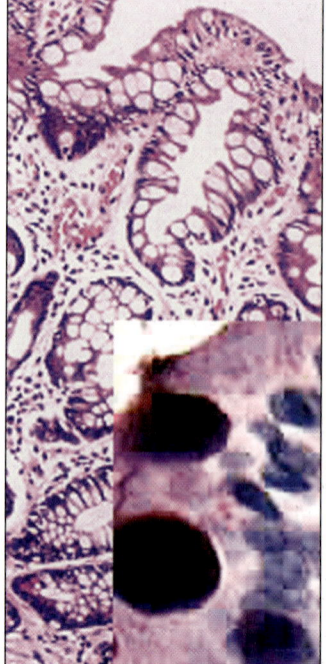

Figure 6.4 Intestinal metaplasia of antral mucosa. Inset shows large goblet cells packed with mucin (shown by Alcian blue staining)

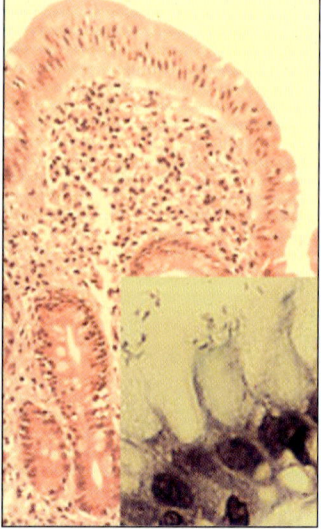

Figure 6.5 Duodenum with gastric metaplasia and mild inflammation. Inset shows *H pylori* adhering to surface epithelial cells

Host

Studies of identical and non-identical twins have shown that host factors are important in determining the outcome of infection. Duodenal ulcer is twice as common in those who are blood group O non-secretors. Studies in the mouse model of *Helicobacter* infection have shown that different strains of mice developed either severe gastritis or hardly any gastritis when infected with the same strain of *Helicobacter*. The genes responsible for the different outcomes are not known, but preliminary evidence suggests that a variety of genes involved in the inflammatory response affect the likelihood of *H pylori* infection progressing to duodenal ulcer disease.

Bacterium

In contrast, some investigators believe that *H pylori* is mainly responsible for disease because gastric mucosal inflammation is always present and fully resolves only when infection is successfully treated. Most strains of *H pylori* can be divided into two distinct phenotypes based on the presence or absence of a vacuolating toxin (Vac A toxin) and the products of the cag pathogenicity island (cagPI), a large chromosomal region that encodes virulence genes and is similar to that found in other enteric pathogens such as *Escherichia coli* and *Salmonella typhi*. People infected with strains of *H pylori* with the cagPI have more severe mucosal damage and are more likely to have duodenal ulcers or gastric cancer.

However, research has not so far identified *H pylori* genes that predispose to either duodenal ulcer or gastric cancer. Furthermore, in developing countries, where *H pylori* infects most of the population, cagPI strains of *H pylori* are present in almost all infected people but only a few develop clinical disease.

Identifying these and other bacterial virulence factors associated with more severe disease may allow screening tests to be developed. These may then permit identification of patients infected with "bad" bacteria so that eradication treatment can be targeted to them.

Environment

Gastric cancer is epidemiologically linked with diets high in salt and low in fresh fruit. Salt may change acid secretion because it suppresses parietal cells, and salty diets cause gastric atrophy. Conversely, the antioxidant vitamins in fresh fruit might protect specialised gastric cells from the reactive oxygen species released by inflammatory cells. A diet high in salt and lacking antioxidant vitamins might thus promote low acid secretion with corpus gastritis. Cigarette smoking strongly predisposes to both duodenal ulcer and gastric cancer.

Time and geographical trends

The factors described above might explain some geographical differences and changes with time in the prevalence of the different upper gastrointestinal diseases. For example, a high prevalence of *H pylori* infection plus a traditional salty diet might explain the high prevalence of gastric cancer in Japan and China. Rates of acid secretion have risen recently in Japan, perhaps because of a fall in the prevalence of *H pylori* or some Westernisation of the diet. In the United Kingdom the replacement of salt with refrigeration to preserve food might have accounted for the rise in the prevalence of duodenal ulcer disease in the middle of this century, as the gastric corpus became healthier and acid secretion higher.

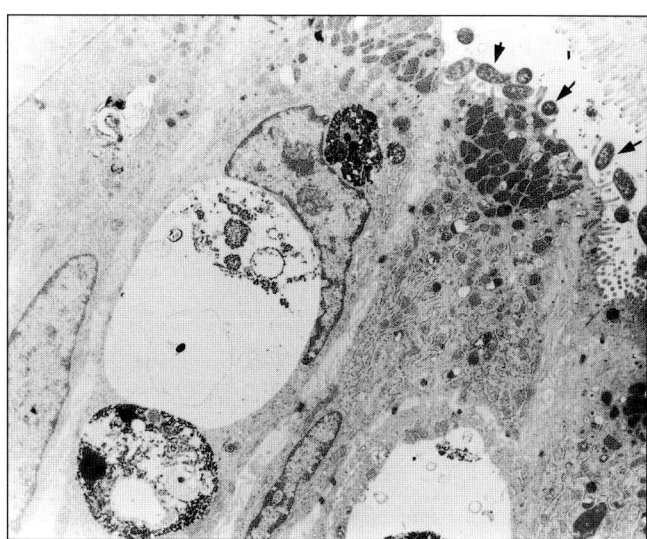

Figure 6.6 Transmission electron micrograph of duodenal gastric metaplasia with *H pylori* attached to the apical surface (arrows)

Box 6.2 Summary points

- Both duodenal ulcer and gastric ulcer are essentially gastric ulcers
- They occur in gastric mucosa in the stomach or in gastric metaplasia mucosa in the duodenum
- The mucosa may be attacked by
  Secretagogues (excess gastrin, histamine, or calcium producing excess of acid)
  Bacteria (*H pylori*)
  Drugs (non-steroidal anti-inflammatory drugs)

Further reading

- Calam J. *Clinicians guide to Helicobacter pylori*. London: Chapman and Hall, 1996
- El-Omar EM, Penman ID, Ardill JES, Chittajallu RS, Howie C, McColl KEL. Helicobacter pylori infection and abnormalities of acid secretion in patients with duodenal ulcer disease. *Gastroenterology* 1995;109:681-91
- Harris AW, Grummett PA, Misiewicz JJ, Baron JH. Eradication of Helicobacter pylori in patients with duodenal ulcers lowers basal and peak acid outputs in response to gastrin releasing peptide and pentagastrin. *Gut* 1996;38:663-7
- Logan RPH, Walker MM, Misiewicz JJ, Gummett PA, Karim QN, Baron JH. Changes in the intragastric distribution of Helicobacter pylori during treatment with omeprazole. *Gut* 1995;36:12-6
- Saponin P, Hyvarinen H, Psoralea M. H pylori corpus gastritis—relation to acid output. *J Physiol Pharmacol* 1996;47:151-9

7 Management of *Helicobacter pylori* infection

Adam Harris, J J Misiewicz

This article discusses the current management of *Helicobacter pylori* infection in patients with dyspepsia with or without endoscopic abnormalities. We take an evidence based approach when possible and consider recent guidelines from national and international bodies pertaining to primary and secondary care.

Duodenal ulcer disease

In patients who are not taking non-steroidal anti-inflammatory drugs (NSAIDs) duodenal ulcer will be due to *H pylori* infection in 95% of cases, and eradication treatment can be prescribed without testing for *H pylori*. If there is any doubt about the diagnosis, such as a possible ulcer crater on a barium meal, endoscopic confirmation of duodenal ulcer and *H pylori* infection should be sought before prescribing treatment.

H pylori eradication treatment, if successful, will be effective in curing the ulcer diathesis regardless of whether a patient is seen at the initial presentation of the disease or at a recurrence. Patients taking long term (maintenance) treatment with H_2 receptor antagonists or proton pump inhibitors should also be offered *H pylori* eradication treatment regardless of whether they are free of symptoms or still experiencing indigestion. In most cases eradication of *H pylori* cures the duodenal ulcer disease, and maintenance treatment can be stopped.

After eradication treatment
Uncomplicated duodenal ulcers heal quickly and completely after eradication of *H pylori*. Further antisecretory treatment, repeat endoscopy, or formal assessment of eradication is not necessary, and one can await the clinical outcome.

Recurrent symptoms indicate either eradication failure or the presence of some other disease. Subsequent management will not be clear unless the outcome of eradication treatment is known, and this is best assessed by a ^{13}C-urea breath test performed more than four weeks after the antimicrobial treatment. Recurrent symptoms after documented *H pylori* eradication are often due to gastro-oesophageal reflux disease, the symptoms of which may be misattributed to duodenal ulcer.

Complicated duodenal ulcer
Complicated duodenal ulcers (such as bleeding or perforated) are associated with appreciable morbidity and mortality, especially in elderly people. Therefore, in patients with complicated duodenal ulcers, eradication of *H pylori* and complete epithelialisation of the ulcer crater need to be confirmed by the ^{13}C-urea breath test and endoscopy, after which maintenance antisecretory treatment can be stopped. The prevalence of *H pylori* infection in patients with complicated duodenal ulcer may be lower than in those with simple duodenal ulcer, and *H pylori* status should therefore be assessed before prescribing eradication treatment.

Duodenal ulcers recur in about 5% of patients initially infected with *H pylori* even after eradication and in the absence of reinfection or use of NSAIDs. Duodenal ulcers are also found occasionally in people not infected with *H pylori*. After exclusion of surreptitious use of ulcerogenic drugs and the rarer causes of duodenal ulcer, such patients need long term maintenance treatment with antisecretory drugs.

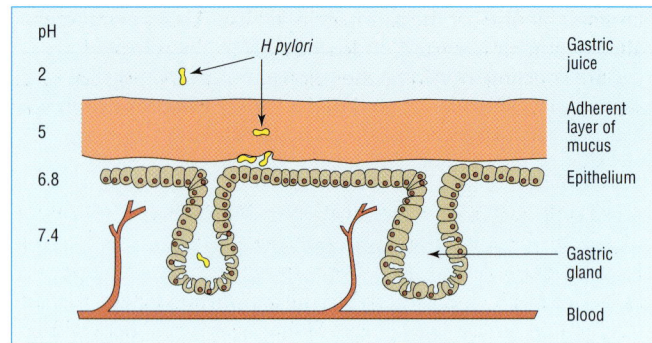

Figure 7.1 Microanatomy of gastric mucosa indicating the pH gradient

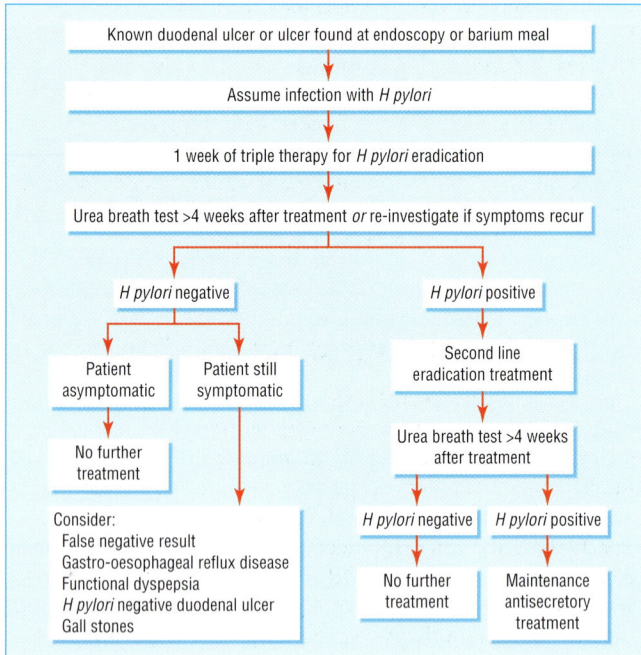

Figure 7.2 Management plan for uncomplicated duodenal ulcer in patients not taking NSAIDs

---

Box 7.1 Causes of duodenal ulcer

Common causes
- *H pylori* infection
- Non-steroidal anti-inflammatory drugs

Rare causes
- Zollinger-Ellison syndrome
- Hypercalcaemia
- Granulomatous diseases (Crohn's disease, sarcoidosis)
- Neoplasia (carcinoma, lymphoma, leiomyoma, leiomyosarcoma)
- Infections (tuberculosis, syphilis, herpes simplex, cytomegalovirus)
- Ectopic pancreatic tissue

Management of *Helicobacter pylori* infection

Gastric ulcer

Diagnosis
The main difference in the management of gastric ulcers from that of duodenal ulcers is the need to exclude malignancy in an apparently benign gastric ulcer. Endoscopy is mandatory, with targeted biopsies of the ulcer rim and base. About eight weeks after treatment is started, endoscopy should be repeated to confirm healing, obtain further biopsies from the original ulcer site, and if clinically indicated ascertain *H pylori* infection status.

Treatment
As with duodenal ulcer, eradication of *H pylori* leads to healing of gastric ulcer and markedly decreases the incidence of relapse. Eradication of *H pylori* also seems to reduce the complications associated with gastric ulcer, but the supporting evidence is less strong than for duodenal ulcer. Maintenance treatment with antisecretory drugs should therefore be started after successful eradication of *H pylori* in those patients with gastric ulcer who have a history of haemorrhage or perforation until complete healing of the ulcer is confirmed at endoscopy.

Ulcers associated with *H pylori* and NSAIDs
Most gastric ulcers associated with *H pylori* infection or with use of NSAIDs occur in elderly women. Despite several studies, no clearly defined guidelines have emerged. NSAIDs and *H pylori* seem to be independent risk factors for increased risk of gastrointestinal bleeding. If a patient infected with *H pylori* has ulceration then *H pylori* should be eradicated before treatment with NSAIDs is started. There is no evidence that *H pylori* eradication relieves NSAID induced dyspepsia.

Gastro-oesophageal reflux disease

The interaction between *H pylori*, gastro-oesophageal reflux disease (GORD), and treatment with antisecretory drugs is extremely complex and highly contentious. Epidemiological studies have shown that the prevalence of *H pylori* infection is no higher in patients with GORD than in healthy controls matched for age and sex. Indeed, *H pylori* infection may be less common in patients with GORD, particularly those with more severe (erosive) disease, suggesting that the bacterium may have a protective role, perhaps by producing corpus gastritis and thus decreasing the output of acid. Moreover, proton pump inhibitors used to treat GORD seem to be more effective at suppressing acid and healing oesophagitis in the presence of *H pylori*. After eradication of the bacterium, patients with GORD may require higher doses and longer duration of proton pump inhibitor treatment.

However, patients with GORD and *H pylori* infection who need prolonged treatment with standard doses of proton pump inhibitors may be at increased risk of developing atrophic gastritis. It is well recognised that chronic atrophic pangastritis is associated with increased risk of proximal gastric adenocarcinoma. During profound acid suppression with proton pump inhibitors, *H pylori* infection spreads from the antrum to the gastric body and fundus and causes a chronic active pangastritis that, with time, may progress to atrophic gastritis. The actual lifetime risk of subsequent gastric cancer is unknown and needs to be evaluated against the potentially detrimental effects of eradicating *H pylori* infection in patients with GORD. Further studies are needed before these contradictory considerations can be resolved.

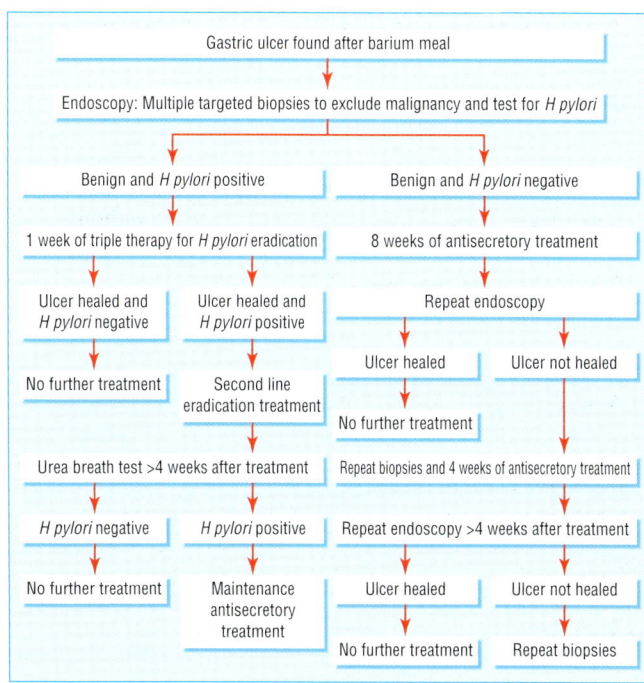

Figure 7.3 Management plan for gastric ulcer

Box 7.2 Causes of gastric ulcer
- *H pylori* infection
- Non-steroidal anti-inflammatory drugs
- Neoplasia (carcinoma, lymphoma, leiomyosarcoma)
- Stress
- Crohn's disease
- Infections (herpes simplex, cytomegalovirus)

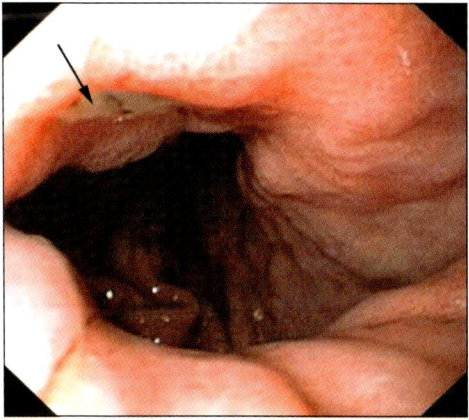

Figure 7.4 Benign gastric ulcer (arrow) in upper part of stomach

Proton pump inhibitors + *H pylori* infection increases atrophic gastritis	Proved?
H pylori eradication reduces efficacy of proton pump inhibitors and H$_2$ receptor antagonists	Relevant?
Barrett's oesophagus and GORD are risk factors for oesophageal cancer	Important?
H pylori pangastritis may protect against Barrett's oesophagus and GORD	Important?
H pylori may cause reflux	True?

Figure 7.5 Interactions between *H pylori*, GORD, and antisecretory drugs

ABC of the Upper Gastrointestinal Tract

Functional dyspepsia

In the absence of NSAID treatment, about 60% of young patients (<45 years old) with dyspepsia have functional dyspepsia, about 25% have GORD, and 15% have peptic ulcer disease. Although the evidence unequivocally supports *H pylori* eradication in peptic ulcer disease, the role of *H pylori* in functional dyspepsia and the evidence to support its treatment are much less clear.

Asymptomatic *H pylori* infection

This presentation is becoming more common because of the increasing use of commercial, non-invasive tests for *H pylori*. A positive test often causes concern about the risk of developing stomach cancer; but we don't know when *H pylori* has to be eradicated to prevent the progression to cancer, and there is no evidence yet that eradication of *H pylori* decreases this risk.

H pylori eradication treatment

The aim of treating *H pylori* is to eradicate the organism from the stomach. Eradication is defined as negative tests for the bacterium four weeks or longer after treatment has finished. Premature assessments may give false negative results because of temporary clearance or suppression of *H pylori*. The best test to confirm eradication is the ^{13}C-urea breath test. The recently described stool antigen test may be an alternative in future. "Near patient tests" or laboratory based blood serology tests are not suitable because antibody titres take at least six months to decrease.

Treatment of *H pylori* is difficult because of the rapid development of resistance to antibacterial drugs, especially to nitroimidazoles, which occurs more commonly in women and patients from developing countries because of previous treatment for gynaecological infections or infective diarrhoeas. Resistance to clarithromycin may occur after failed treatment or after use of this drug for other indications such as respiratory tract infections. Resistance to antibiotics other than nitroimidazoles can also develop but is less common

Low dose triple therapy—The most overall effective *H pylori* eradication regimens reported to date combine a proton pump inhibitor with two of the following—amoxicillin, clarithromycin, or a nitroimidazole—for a week. There are few side effects (the commonest being nausea, diarrhoea, and taste disturbance). Results from large randomised controlled trials have shown *H pylori* eradication in about 90% of patients.

Ranitidine-bismuth-citrate has been developed specifically for treating *H pylori* infection. It retains both the antisecretory and antibacterial properties of the parent compounds but achieves acceptable eradication rates only when used as an alternative to a proton pump inhibitor in combination with clarithromycin and either metronidazole or amoxicillin for a week.

Quadruple therapy—Classic bismuth based triple therapy is more effective when coprescribed with a proton pump inhibitor (80-90% *H pylori* eradication). Efficacy is highly dependent on compliance with the complicated regimen, and there are numerous side effects. It is best reserved for use by hospital specialists to treat patients in whom triple therapy has failed.

What to tell patients?

There has been much discussion of *H pylori* in the media, and many patients are aware of its ulcerogenic and carcinogenic potential and may request antibacterial treatment if they are found to be infected. Eradication treatment is of proved benefit

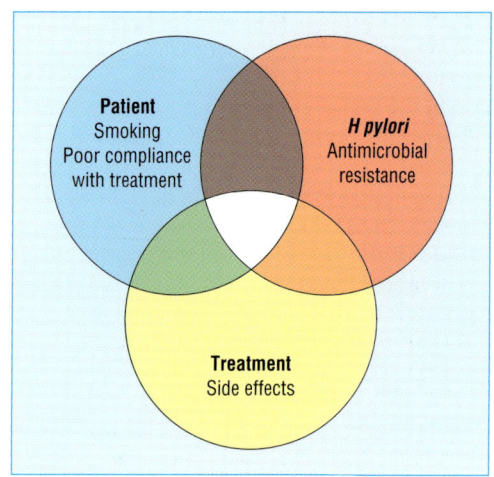

Figure 7.6 Possible reasons for failure of *H pylori* eradication

Box 7.3 Risk factors for nitroimidazole resistance in *H pylori*
- Previous use of nitroimidazoles, such as for gynaecological infections, infective diarrhoeas
- Failed eradication of *H pylori* with treatment regimen containing a nitroimidazole
- Urban or inner city areas
- Patients born in developing countries

Table 7.1 Low dose triple therapy for *H pylori* eradication

	Proton pump inhibitor twice daily	Proton pump inhibitor twice daily
Treatment	Amoxicillin 1 g twice daily	Clarithromycin 250 mg twice daily
	Clarithromycin 500 mg twice daily	Metronidazole 400 mg twice daily
Duration	1 week	
Side effects	Nausea, diarrhoea, taste disturbances	
Eradication	90%	90% in MSS 75% in MRS

MSS = metronidazole sensitive strain of *H pylori*. MRS = metronidazole resistant strain of *H pylori*

Table 7.2 Quadruple therapy for *H pylori* eradication

Treatment	Proton pump inhibitor once or twice daily
	Colloidal bismuth citrate 120 mg four times daily
	Tetracycline 500 mg four times daily
	Metronidazole 400 mg four times daily
Duration	1 week
Side effects	Commonly nausea, diarrhoea, taste disturbances
Eradication	>75% in MRS >90% in MSS

MRS = metronidazole resistant strain of *H pylori*. MSS = metronidazole sensitive strain of *H pylori*

only in patients with duodenal or gastric ulcer associated with *H pylori* infection. At present there is no evidence to suggest that screening and treating patients without risk factors will prevent gastric cancer. The risk of transmission to partners is low in adults, and treatment of the entire family is not warranted.

Counselling patients
Whatever treatment is chosen, patients need careful counselling. The reasons for embarking on the treatment and the importance of compliance despite possible side effects need to be emphasised, and the possible side effects must be carefully discussed. The need for good compliance needs special attention, as it is crucial to the success of treatment.

First line treatment—In areas with a low prevalence (<30%) of metronidazole resistant strains of *H pylori* one week of low dose triple therapy consisting of a proton pump inhibitor, metronidazole, and clarithromycin is currently recommended. Patients' compliance with treatment is likely to be good because of twice daily dosing and few side effects. If metronidazole resistance is likely a proton pump inhibitor in combination with amoxicillin and clarithromycin given for one week is preferable.

Second line treatment—After a proved failure with a treatment containing metronidazole, a patient is likely to be colonised by a resistant strain of *H pylori*. In this case a proton pump inhibitor should be given in combination with amoxicillin and clarithromycin for a week, with about 90% success. If *H pylori* eradication is unsuccessful after a treatment containing clarithromycin and the patient is likely to harbour a metronidazole resistant strain of *H pylori*, then either omeprazole in combination with amoxicillin and metronidazole or quadruple therapy are the only logical options, with roughly 75% success.

Summary

Despite a vast amount of research, the only evidence based indications for eradication of *H pylori* are for patients with duodenal ulcer or gastric ulcer who are not taking NSAIDs and for patients with the extremely rare MALT lymphoma. Low dose triple therapy given for one week will cure most patients of their infection: failures are due to bacterial resistance or poor compliance. The importance of *H pylori* in NSAID associated ulceration is uncertain. Although *H pylori* is strongly associated with gastric cancer, there is no proof that eradication treatment decreases an individual's risk of that disease.

Table 7.3 Indications for *H pylori* eradication treatment

Diagnosis	Evidence based indication
Duodenal ulcers not due to NSAIDs	Yes
Gastric ulcers not due to NSAIDs	Yes
Duodenal or gastric ulcers due to NSAIDs	No
Functional dyspepsia	Unknown or no
Gastro-oesophageal reflux disease	Unknown or no
Gastric cancer	Unknown or no
MALT lymphoma	Yes

NSAID = non-steroidal anti-inflammatory drug

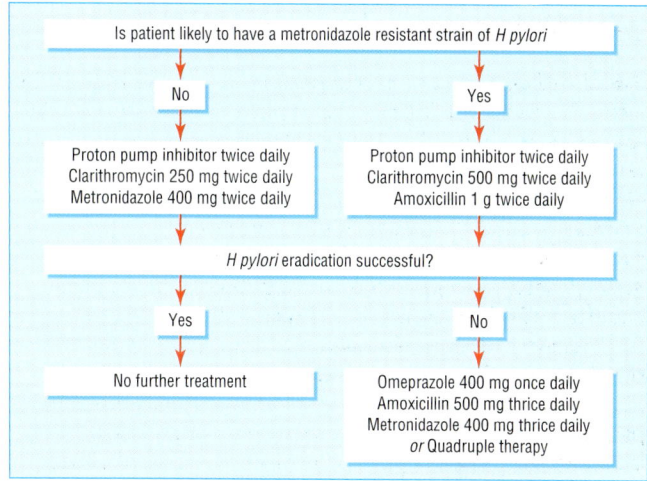

Figure 7.7 Choosing a treatment regimen for *H pylori* eradication

The endoscopic image of benign gastric ulcer is reproduced with permission of Gastrolab Image Gallery.

8 Indigestion and non-steroidal anti-inflammatory drugs

J M Seager, C J Hawkey

Non-steroidal anti-inflammatory drugs (NSAIDs) are usually thought to pose a dilemma for doctors wishing to prescribe them. Their anti-inflammatory and analgesic properties have led to their widespread use for rheumatoid and (much more commonly) other conditions often regarded as more trivial. However they are ulcerogenic to the stomach and duodenum and lead to a threefold to 10-fold increase in ulcer complications, hospitalisation, and death from ulcer disease.[1]

In fact, the dilemma is more complex than whether potentially life threatening drugs should be used to manage conditions that are uncomfortable but not in themselves life threatening. There is growing evidence that NSAIDs have other incidental benefits. The only study to investigate overall life expectancy with drug use found non-significant trends towards enhanced rather than reduced life expectancy. Aspirin has benefits in preventing cardiovascular disease and probably cancer that seem to far outweigh the hazards of gastrointestinal ulceration. Limited evidence suggests that these benefits may be shared by other NSAIDs.

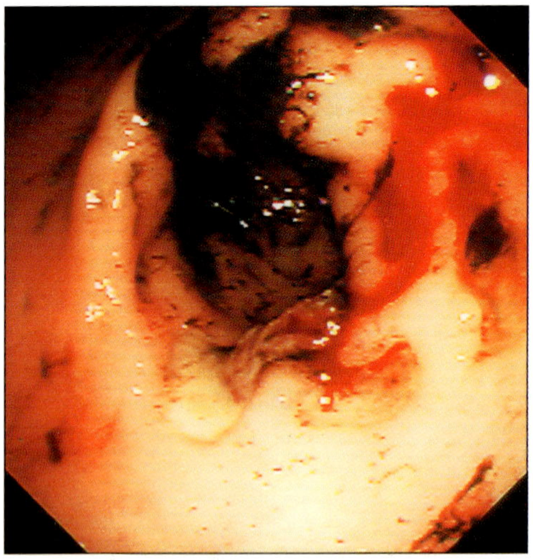

NSAID use

About 24 million prescriptions a year are written for NSAIDs in the United Kingdom. Half of these are given to patients over the age of 60. At any one time about 15% of elderly people are taking an NSAID. Average prescribing rates are calculated to be 426 scripts per 1000 population per year.

Less than 10% of NSAIDs used in the community seem to be for rheumatoid arthritis, and less than half for any form of arthritis. They are widely used for acute soft tissue injury and more chronically for undiagnosed pains in the back and elsewhere. Chronic use is more common in elderly than younger patients, and prophylactic use of aspirin, mostly in relatively low doses, for cardiovascular events is increasing, amounting to 9.5% of a relatively elderly population.

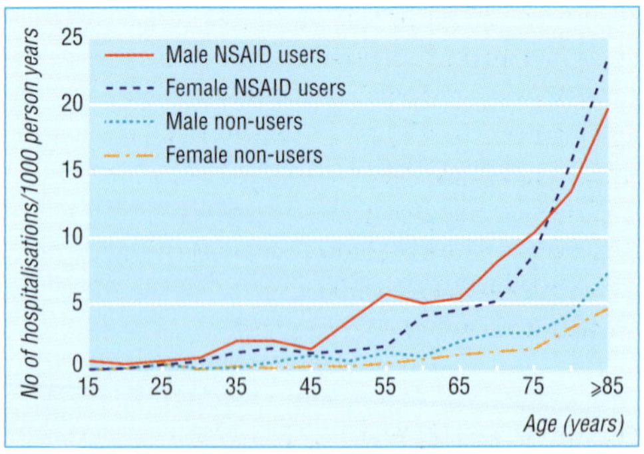

Gastrointestinal toxicity of NSAIDs

NSAIDs are important in causing both (non-ulcer) dyspepsia and ulcers (often silent and presenting with a complication). The unreliability of dyspepsia as a pointer to ulceration underlies many of the problems of managing patients taking NSAIDs.

Within 90 minutes of taking 300 mg or 600 mg of aspirin, nearly everyone develops acute injury consisting of intramucosal petechiae and erosions. Non-aspirin NSAIDs cause less florid acute injury, but endoscopic studies show that about 20% of those taking non-aspirin NSAIDs or aspirin at anti-inflammatory doses chronically have a gastric or duodenal ulcer. Many patients who start NSAIDs will not be able to continue because of drug associated dyspepsia.

Ulcers probably form and heal spontaneously in most NSAID users and usually cause little harm. However, about once in every 50-100 patient years, ulcer bleeding or perforation develops that requires hospitalisation.[2] As a consequence, probably at least 1200 patients die each year in the United Kingdom.[1]

Figure 8.1 Three ulcers (one bleeding) in the gastric antrum caused by NSAIDs. Such ulcer complications are estimated to cause up to 16 500 deaths each year in the United States and 2000 deaths a year in Britain

Figure 8.2 Hospitalisations due to complications associated with NSAID use are a problem in elderly patients

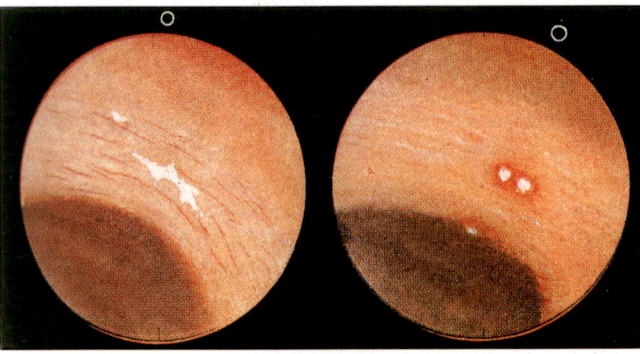

Figure 8.3 In 1938 Douthwaite and Lintott provided the first endoscopic evidence that aspirin caused gastric mucosal damage. Images show gastric antrum before (left) and after (right) administration of aspirin (reproduced from Douthwaite AH, Lintott JAM. *Lancet* 1938;ii:1222-5)

Who is at particular risk?

Risk factors for gastroduodenal ulcer complications are now fairly well defined. Most patients with NSAID associated ulcer complications are elderly. This is because elderly people have a higher background prevalence of ulcer problems, are more likely to receive NSAIDs, and are probably more sensitive to them. A history of ulcers (whether or not associated with NSAIDs) is a further risk factor.

A meta-analysis of recent studies shows that ibuprofen (≤1200 mg/day) is associated with a lower level of risk than other NSAIDs, whereas others such as azapropazone and piroxicam are associated with a higher risk.[3] These differences probably relate at least in part to effective dose, since doses of ibuprofen greater than 1200 mg carry risks similar to those with other NSAIDs.[3] Among NSAIDs in general, risks rise steadily with dose.[3]

As would be expected, the risk of ulcer bleeding is much higher if patients taking NSAIDs also receive warfarin. Interestingly, use of corticosteroids has been shown fairly consistently to magnify the risk of ulcer complications, to the extent that ulcers associated with NSAIDs and steroid may account for the probably incorrect belief that corticosteroids were themselves ulcerogenic.

Box 8.1 Risk factors for gastrointestinal complications occurring with NSAIDs

Patient related factors
- Age >60 years
- History of ulcer disease

Drug related factors
- Use of relatively toxic NSAID
- High dose of NSAID (or two NSAIDs used concurrently)
- Concurrent use of anticoagulant
- Concurrent use of corticosteroid

Uncertain or possible risk factors
- Duration of NSAID treatment
- Female
- Underlying rheumatic disease
- Cardiovascular disease
- *Helicobacter pylori* infection
- Smoking
- Alcohol consumption

Managing patients taking NSAIDs

Management of patients who need to take NSAIDs should be based more on assessment of risk than on clinical, laboratory, or endoscopic investigation. NSAID use should be avoided in patients with two or three of the risk factors for ulcer complications, or if this is not possible they should receive prophylactic treatment.

Although development of dyspepsia soon after starting an NSAID may preclude its use and can sometimes lead to discovery of a previously silent ulcer, NSAID associated dyspepsia is generally a poor guide to the presence of an ulcer. Development of anaemia or new onset dyspepsia can identify NSAID associated ulcers, but upper gastrointestinal investigation is often negative and reliance on these signs will miss most ulcers, which most commonly present with complications on a relatively silent background.

Available drugs to treat ulcers

Preclinical studies in animals and humans suggest that two components contribute to development of NSAID associated ulcers. Firstly, inhibition of prostaglandin synthesis, by impairing mucosal defences, leads to erosive breach of the epithelial barrier. Secondly, acid peptic attack deepens this into frank ulceration, and pH is also an important determinant of passive NSAID absorption and trapping in the mucosa. Preventive treatment aimed at either mucosal defence or acid attack is available.

Misoprostol is a stable analogue of prostaglandin E₁. Several studies show that it prevents acute gastric injury by a wide variety of agents including NSAIDs. In doses of 400-800 μg daily misoprostol prevents gastric (and probably duodenal) ulcers. A large study has shown it to reduce the incidence of hospitalisation for NSAID associated gastrointestinal complications.[2] Unfortunately, as a prostaglandin, it causes diarrhoea, abdominal cramps, and reflux at the doses necessary to protect against NSAID associated ulcers.

Acid suppressing drugs—Normal doses of H₂ antagonists have relatively little affect on acute aspirin and NSAID associated injury in animals and in humans. High doses of H₂ antagonists

Table 8.1 Comparative toxicity of NSAIDs for gastrointestinal complications*

Drug	No of studies	Pooled relative risk (95% CI)†	P value (heterogenicity)
Ibuprofen	NA	1.0	NA
Fenoprofen	2	1.6 (1.0 to 2.5)	0.310
Aspirin	6	1.6 (1.3 to 2.0)	0.685
Diclofenac	8	1.8 (1.4 to 2.3)	0.778
Sulindac	5	2.1 (1.6 to 2.7)	0.685
Diflunisal	2	2.2 (1.2 to 4.1)	0.351
Naproxen	10	2.2 (1.7 to 2.9)	0.131
Indometacin	11	2.4 (1.9 to 3.1)	0.488
Tolmetin	2	3.0 (1.8 to 4.9)	0.298
Piroxicam	10	3.8 (2.7 to 5.2)	0.087
Ketoprofen	7	4.2 (2.7 to 6.4)	0.258
Azapropazone	2	9.2 (4.0 to 21.0)	0.832

*Adapted from Henry et al.[3]
†Relative to ibuprofen.

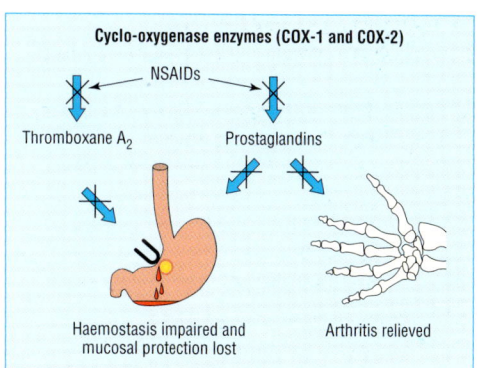

Figure 8.4 Inhibition of cyclo-oxygenase enzymes by NSAIDs relieves inflammation and pain but also removes mucosal protection of gastric epithelium

ABC of the Upper Gastrointestinal Tract

and normal doses of proton pump inhibitors are protective, and long term studies have shown them to prevent both gastric and duodenal ulcers. There have been no randomised studies of the effect of acid suppression on NSAID associated complications, although indirect evidence from epidemiology is encouraging.

Choice of treatment

Patients with NSAID associated ulcers
If patients present with ulcers NSAIDs should be stopped if possible since they retard healing. For patients who need to continue taking NSAIDs, large comparative studies have shown that omeprazole 20 mg daily results in faster healing of gastric and duodenal ulcers than ranitidine 150 mg twice daily[4] or misoprostol 200 µg four times daily and is better tolerated than misoprostol.

Subsequent prevention of relapse
Studies have shown that, once healing is achieved, NSAID associated ulcer relapse can be retarded by use of omeprazole, misoprostol, or high dose famotidine.[4] These comparative studies—based on preventing the development of ulcers, multiple erosions, or moderate to severe dyspepsia—have shown overall higher efficacy for omeprazole 20 mg daily than misoprostol 200 µg twice daily or ranitidine 150 mg twice daily.[4] In these studies omeprazole protected against ulcers, both gastric and particularly duodenal, and erosions. Misoprostol was associated with the same rate of duodenal ulcer formation as placebo but was particularly effective in preventing multiple erosions. In these studies the site of the initial lesion was a strong predictor of the site of subsequent relapse.

NSAID users without ulcers
Many studies have shown that misoprostol can inhibit ulcer development in such patients, as can famotidine 40 mg twice daily and omeprazole. These drugs have not been compared for relative effectiveness in this group of patients.

Practical prescribing
Patients presenting with gastric or duodenal ulcers who need to continue taking NSAIDs should be treated with omeprazole 20 mg daily or another proton pump inhibitor until the ulcer heals. Although omeprazole is the only proton pump inhibitor to have been studied in large scale trials, its benefits are probably a class effect. Patients with multiple erosions instead may be better served by misoprostol.

Overall, subsequent maintenance treatment is likely to be more effective and better tolerated with a proton pump inhibitor than misoprostol. Recognition that the site and nature of the original lesion is a strong predictor of the site and nature of relapse can aid management.

For patients who present with duodenal ulcers a proton pump inhibitor is an appropriate maintenance treatment. For patients with multiple erosions misoprostol is appropriate if tolerated. On current data there is little to choose between proton pump inhibitors and misoprostol with regard to efficacy in preventing gastric ulcers, but proton pump inhibitors are better tolerated.

Role of *Helicobacter pylori* eradication

This is an extremely controversial topic. One study, of patients starting NSAIDs (naproxen) for the first time without a history of dyspepsia or ulceration, showed that eradication of *H pylori*

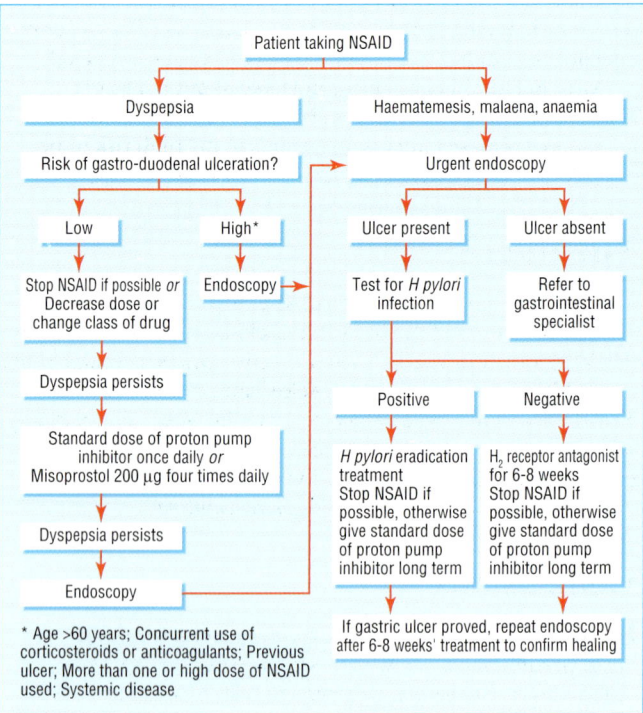

Figure 8.5 Algorithm for managing gastrointestinal side effects of NSAIDs

---

Box 8.2 Side effects of NSAIDs
- Dyspepsia
- Oesophagitis
- Oesophageal strictures
- Gastric and duodenal petechiae, erosions, ulceration, bleeding, and perforation
- Type C gastritis
- Small and large bowel ulceration, bleeding, and perforation
- Exacerbation of colitis

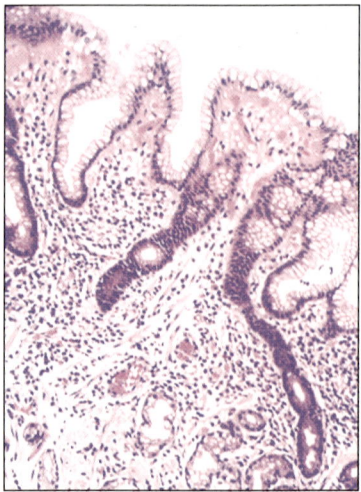

Figure 8.6 Chemical (type C) gastritis showing oedema and mild chronic inflammation of lamina propria and vertical smooth muscle fibres and slight foveolar hyperplasia. Contrast with *H pylori* induced gastritis, which has a marked neutrophil infiltrate in the lamina propria and deeper gastric glands

substantially reduced the rate of gastric ulcer formation at two months. In another study, of patients who had previously had ulcers or moderate to severe dyspepsia, *H pylori* eradication did not influence outcome at six months. Finally, although omeprazole is effective prophylaxis in patients without *H pylori* infection, it is more effective in those who remain infected.[4]

Most doctors, feeling uncomfortable about persistent *H pylori* infection, eradicate it in NSAID users. In our view this is irrational if these patients are at sufficiently high risk to be candidates for co-treatment with acid suppressing drugs.

The future

A new generation of less toxic NSAIDs is probably imminent. Specific inhibitors of the inducible cyclo-oxygenase-2 enzyme (COX-2), which probably leave protective gastric prostaglandins uninhibited, are now available. Meloxicam, another recent NSAID, is well tolerated. Whether this is because it is a partially selective COX-2 inhibitor or because tested doses are low is uncertain. Other developments include NSAIDs that donate cytoprotective nitric oxide to the gastric mucosa.[5]

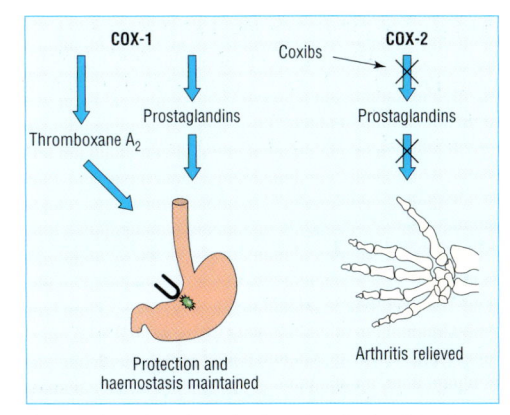

Figure 8.7 Rofecoxib and celecoxib, selective COX-2 inhibitors, can relieve pain and inflammation without risking gastric ulceration

Conclusions

Currently, there is a wide range of views about what is an appropriate level of NSAID prescribing and no simple, all embracing resolution. In patients with risk factors for gastrointestinal complications the side effects of NSAIDs may outweigh all benefits. For such patients, omeprazole and misoprostol can provide effective protection, and the choice is between patients' generally poor tolerance of misoprostol and the higher costs of omeprazole. Finally, a growing concern is the correct management of low dose aspirin used for cardiovascular protection, and no patient studies have specifically investigated this.

Box 8.3 NSAID protection strategies
- Use lowest possible doses of NSAIDs
- Use safer NSAIDs
  Low toxicity NSAIDs
  COX-2 inhibitors
- Use NSAID prophylaxis
  Proton pump inhibitors
  Misoprostil

---

1 Hawkey CJ. Non steroidal anti-inflammatory drugs and peptic ulcers: facts and figures multiply, but do they add up? *BMJ* 1990;300:278-84.
2 Silverstein FE, Graham DY, Senior JR, Davies HW, Struthers BJ, Bittman RM, et al. Misoprostol reduces serious gastrointestinal complications in patients with rheumatoid arthritis receiving nonsteroidal anti-inflammatory drugs. *Ann Intern Med* 1995;123:241-9.
3 Henry D, Lim LL-Y, Garcia Rodriguez LA, Perez Gutthann S, Carson JL, Griffin M, et al. Variability in risk of gastrointestinal complications with individual non-steroidal anti-inflammatory drugs: results of a collaborative meta-analysis. *BMJ* 1996;312:1563-6.
4 Yeomans ND, Tulassay Z, Juhasz L, Racz I, Howard JM, van Rensburg CJ, et al, for the ASTRONAUT Study Group. A comparison of omeprazole and ranitidine for treating and preventing ulcers associated with non steroidal anti inflammatory drugs. *N Engl J Med* 1998;338:719-26.
5 Hawkey CJ. Future treatments for arthritis—new NSAIDs, NO-NSAIDs or no NSAIDs? *Gastroenterology* 1995;109:614-6.

9 Upper gastrointestinal haemorrhage

Helen J Dallal, K R Palmer

Acute upper gastrointestinal haemorrhage accounts for about 2500 hospital admissions each year in the United Kingdom. The annual incidence varies from 47 to 116 per 100 000 of the population and is higher in socioeconomically deprived areas.

Although hospital mortality has not improved over 50 years and remains at about 10%, older patients who have advanced cardiovascular, respiratory, or cerebrovascular disease that puts them at increased risk of death now comprise a much higher proportion of cases. Many patients' bleeding is associated with use of non-steroidal anti-inflammatory drugs, but there is no evidence that prognosis is worse in patients who are taking these drugs than in those who are not.

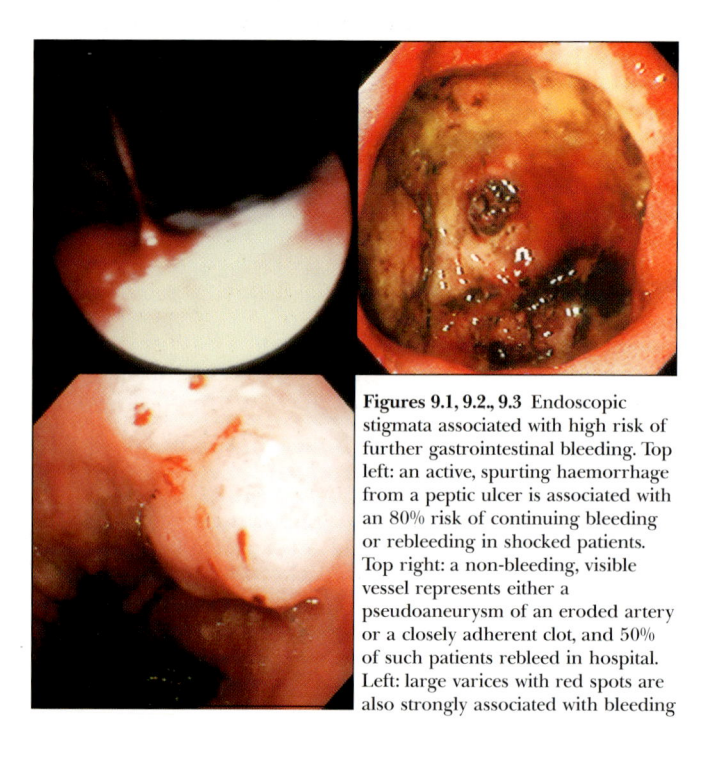

Presentation of bleeding

All patients who develop acute gastrointestinal bleeding need urgent assessment. Almost all should be admitted as an emergency to hospital. Only a small minority of young, fit patients who have self limiting bleeding can be managed as outpatients, but even those need urgent investigation. Patients who present with haematemesis tend to have more severe bleeding than those who present with melaena alone.

At the initial assessment it is important to define factors that have prognostic importance. The main factors predicting death include increasing age, comorbidity, and endoscopic findings. Mortality is extremely low in patients under 40 years old but thereafter increases steeply with advancing age. Patients who have severe comorbidity—particularly renal insufficiency, hepatic failure, or disseminated malignancy—have a poor prognosis. Hospital admission may be precipitated by gastrointestinal bleeding in many of these patients, and death is often due to disease progression rather than to bleeding.

A risk assessment score has been developed based on the outcome of 4185 patients with acute gastrointestinal bleeding admitted to hospitals in England.[1] A series of independent risk factors were scored, and the total score accurately predicts outcome. Patients who score 2 or less have a mortality of 0.1% and a rebleeding rate of 4.3%, but a score in excess of 8 is associated with a 41% mortality and rebleeding rate of 42.1%.

Patients who develop acute upper gastrointestinal haemorrhage after hospitalisation for other serious illness have a much worse prognosis than those who are admitted because of bleeding, with a mortality of about 30%. Endoscopic findings of active, spurting haemorrhage; a non-bleeding blood vessel visible within an ulcer; and red spots on large varices are associated with risk of further bleeding. The absence of these endoscopic stigmata indicates little chance of rebleeding and early discharge from hospital.

Causes of bleeding

The commonest cause of upper gastrointestinal haemorrhage is peptic ulcer. A history of proved ulcer or ulcer-like dyspepsia is absent in about 20% of cases. In these patients consumption of aspirin or non-steroidal anti-inflammatory drugs is common. Infection with *Helicobacter pylori* is less prevalent in bleeding ulcers than in uncomplicated ulcers. Severe ulcer bleeding is due to erosion of the artery by the ulcer, and the severity of bleeding depends on the size of the ulcer and the size of the arterial defect. Bleeding from a defect greater than 1 mm in

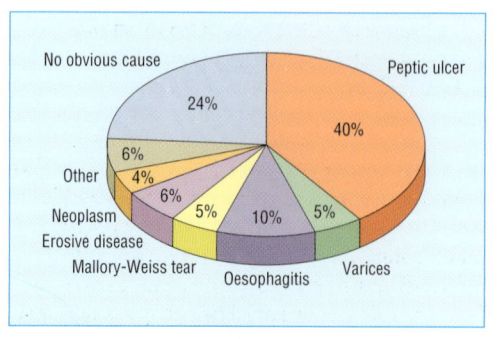

Figures 9.1, 9.2., 9.3 Endoscopic stigmata associated with high risk of further gastrointestinal bleeding. Top left: an active, spurting haemorrhage from a peptic ulcer is associated with an 80% risk of continuing bleeding or rebleeding in shocked patients. Top right: a non-bleeding, visible vessel represents either a pseudoaneurysm of an eroded artery or a closely adherent clot, and 50% of such patients rebleed in hospital. Left: large varices with red spots are also strongly associated with bleeding

---

Box 9.1 Risk factors for death after hospital admission for acute upper gastrointestinal haemorrhage

- Advanced age
- Shock on admission (pulse rate > 100 beats/min; systolic blood pressure < 100 mm Hg)
- Comorbidity (particularly hepatic or renal failure and disseminated cancer)
- Diagnosis (worst prognosis for advanced upper gastrointestinal malignancy)
- Endoscopic findings (active, spurting haemorrhage from peptic ulcer; non-bleeding, visible blood vessel; large varices with red spots)
- Rebleeding (increases mortality 10-fold)

Figure 9.4 Causes of acute upper gastrointestinal haemorrhage

Upper gastrointestinal haemorrhage

diameter is unlikely to stop spontaneously and does not respond to endoscopic treatment. Large ulcers arising from the posterior part of the duodenal cap can erode the gastroduodenal artery and provoke brisk bleeding.

Bleeding from gastric erosions, oesophagitis, or vascular malformations usually stops spontaneously and is not usually life threatening. Mallory-Weiss tears are a consequence of retching, and most patients have a history of alcohol misuse, have features of other gastrointestinal disease such as peptic ulcer or gastroenteritis, or have non-gastrointestinal causes of vomiting. Bleeding usually stops spontaneously, although endoscopic haemostatic treatment is sometimes required.

Bleeding from upper gastrointestinal malignancy is not usually severe, and the prognosis is dictated by the stage of the disease. Patients with extensive upper gastrointestinal cancer have a dismal prognosis, but death is not usually a consequence of gastrointestinal haemorrhage but of disease progression.

In any patient with acute gastrointestinal bleeding liver disease should be considered because it requires specific management. Oesophageal varices account for a small proportion of cases but have a disproportionate impact on medical resources. Bleeding is often severe, and other features of liver failure—such as fluid retention, hepatic encephalopathy, renal failure, and sepsis—often develop after the bleed. About a third of patients will die, and prognosis is related to the severity of the underlying liver disease rather than the size of variceal haemorrhage.

Aortoduodenal fistula must be considered in patients who develop profuse bleeding and have undergone aortic aneurysm surgery.

Management of bleeding

Primary care management
Initial resuscitation of shocked patients can be started before hospital admission. Intravenous access should be obtained, and infusion of a crystalloid started. Oxygen should be given. Management in primary care is limited, and the priority is to arrange early admission to hospital and to support associated comorbidity, such as that of angina or chest disease.

Hospital management
Resuscitation
The first priority is to support the circulation rather than to identify the source of bleeding. Endoscopy is undertaken once resuscitation has been achieved. At least one large bore cannula is inserted into a substantial vein. When the pulse rate is more than 100 beats/min or the systolic blood pressure falls below 100 mm Hg, infusion with a crystalloid such as normal saline is started. The rate of infusion depends on the severity of shock. A recent meta-analysis showed that crystalloids (such as normal saline) should be used rather than colloids (such as dextrans). If blood transfusion is required the aim is to maintain a haemoglobin concentration of 100 g/l. In patients with suspected liver disease the use of normal saline should be avoided because of the risk of precipitating ascites.

Endoscopy
After resuscitation, endoscopy is undertaken. In most cases this is done electively on the next available routine list but within 24 hours of admission. Only a minority of profusely bleeding patients need "out of hours" emergency endoscopy.

On-call endoscopists must be experienced and be able to apply a range of endoscopic treatments. Endoscopy is necessary to define the cause of bleeding, provide prognostic information, and to apply haemostatic treatment.

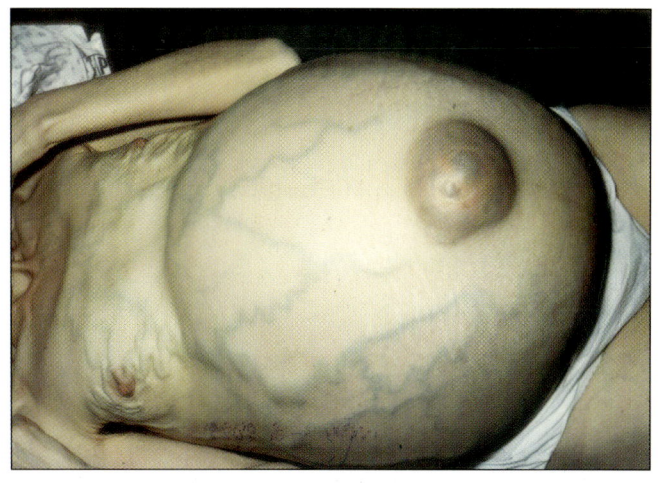

Figure 9.5 Gross ascites and distended abdominal veins in advanced cirrhosis

Box 9.2 Alert for features of liver disease
- Ascites
- Splenomegaly
- Jaundice
- Fluid retention
- Alcohol misuse

Box 9.3 Blood tests on admission to hospital

Haemoglobin concentration—May be normal during the acute stages until haemodilution occurs

Urea and electrolyte concentrations—Elevated blood urea suggests severe bleeding

Cross match for transfusion—Two units of blood are sufficient unless bleeding is extreme. If transfusion not needed urgently group the blood and save the serum

Liver function tests

Prothrombin time

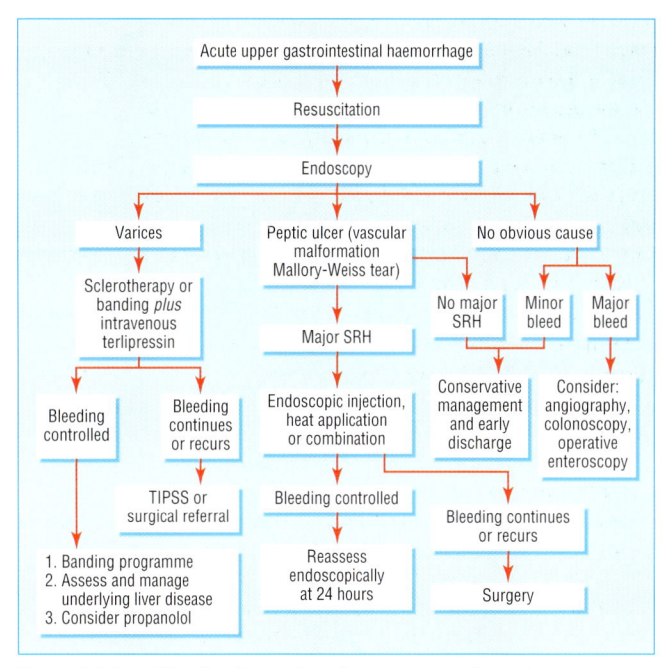

Figure 9.6 Algorithm for diagnosis and management of upper gastrointestinal bleeding (SRH=stigmata of recent haemorrhage, TIPPS=transjugular intrahepatic portosystemic shunt)

ABC of the Upper Gastrointestinal Tract

Diagnosis—It is difficult to prove that diagnostic endoscopy improves outcome, but it is clearly important to define a precise diagnosis in order to plan treatment.

Prognosis—Endoscopic stigmata are extremely useful in defining risk of further bleeding.

Treatment—A range of endoscopic treatments can be administered to patients showing major endoscopic stigmata. Pharmacological, endoscopic, radiological, and surgical treatments are used.

Treatments

Drugs

Non-variceal haemorrhage—There is increasing evidence to support the use of intravenous omeprazole, which in clinical trials reduces the risk of rebleeding and the need for surgical operation. Patients infected with *H pylori* should undergo eradication treatment after haemostasis has been achieved in order to prevent further ulcer complications. One study has shown that tranexamic acid reduces transfusion requirements in patients presenting with non-variceal haemorrhage.

Variceal haemorrhage—Vasoactive drugs (such as terlipressin) reduce bleeding rates but have little impact on survival. If bleeding continues despite this treatment, a modified Sengstaken-Blakemore (Minnesota) tube is inserted. It must be remembered that both vasoactive drugs and the Minnesota tube are temporising measures used to control active bleeding until definitive endoscopic, surgical, or radiological measures are taken. When varices have been obliterated portal pressure is reduced with propanolol at a dose to decrease the pulse rate by 20%. This diminishes the risk of subsequent rebleeding.

Endoscopic treatment

Non-variceal bleeding—A range of endoscopic haemostatic approaches are available. Each has a similar efficacy, but there is evidence that an injection combined with a thermal method is best. Endoscopic treatment fails in about 20% of patients with bleeding ulcers, most often those with large, actively bleeding posterior duodenal ulcers. Endoscopist and surgeon must work together to identify and treat these patients at an early stage.

Varices—When active variceal bleeding is seen at endoscopy, intravariceal injection of a sclerosant (such as 5% ethanolamine, 1% polidoconal, or sodium tetradecyl sulphate) is attempted. An alternative approach is oesophageal band ligation. Banding obliterates varices more efficiently and has few complications, but it may be more difficult to perform in a patient with active bleeding.

Surgery

Surgery is the best way of stopping active ulcer bleeding and preventing rebleeding, but it carries high morbidity and mortality. It is now reserved for cases in which endoscopic treatment has failed. Specific protocols defining indications for a surgical operation are necessary.

Surgical treatment for acute variceal bleeding, including oesophageal transection with devascularisation and porto-caval shunt, is rarely done because of unacceptable mortality. It has been replaced by TIPPS (transjugular intrahepatic portosystemic shunt). However, both interventions may precipitate encephalopathy.

1 Rockall TA, Logan RF, Devlin HB, Northfield TC. Risk assessment after acute upper gastrointestinal haemorrhage. *Gut* 1996;38:316-21.

Box 9.4 Endoscopic treatment for non-variceal bleeding

Thermal
- Heater probe
- Multipolar electrocoagulation

Injection
- Adrenaline (1:10000 to 1:100000)
- Alcohol (98%)
- Sclerosants (ethanolamine, 1% polidoconal)
- Procoagulants (thrombin, fibrin glue)

Mechanical
- Clips
- Sutures
- Staples

Combination

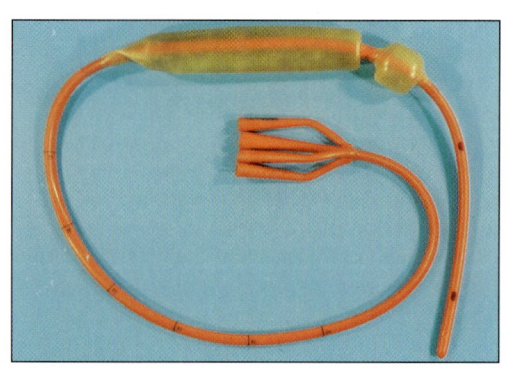

Figure 9.7 Minnesota tube

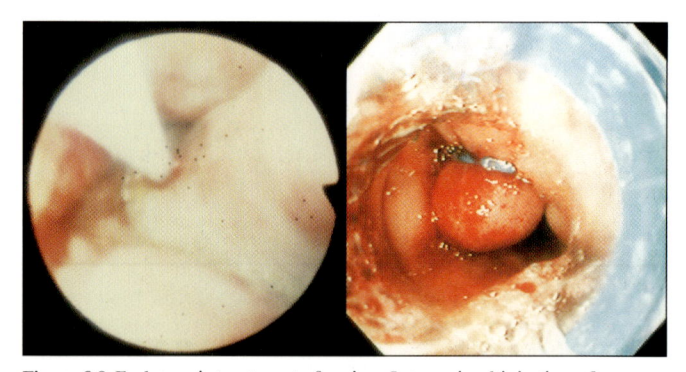

Figure 9.8 Endoscopic treatment of varices. Intravariceal injection of sclerosant (left) and band ligation of oesophageal varices (right)

Box 9.5 Indications for surgical operation for peptic ulcer bleeding

- Active bleeding unresponsive to endoscopic haemostasis
  Profuse bleeding preventing endoscopic visualisation and treatment
  Bleeding continues despite application of endoscopic treatment
- Endoscopically proved rebleeding despite technically successful endoscopic treatment
  Patients at low risk of death, after two unsuccessful attempts at endoscopic treatment
  High risk patients, after one failure of endoscopic haemostasis

10 Indigestion: When is it functional?

Nicholas J Talley, Nghi Phung, Jamshid S Kalantar

Patients often complain of indigestion, but what do they mean? Indigestion is an old English word that means lack of adequate digestion, but patients and doctors interpret this in different ways. Many patients mean heartburn or acid regurgitation, the classic symptoms of gastro-oesophageal reflux disease. Some describe belching, abdominal rumblings, or even bad breath as indigestion. Others mean pain localised to the epigastrium or a non-painful discomfort in the upper abdomen which may be described as fullness, bloating, or an inability to finish a normal meal (early satiety). Dyspepsia is best restricted to mean pain or discomfort centred in the upper abdomen.

There are many causes of dyspepsia, but at least two thirds of patients have no structural or biochemical explanation for their symptoms. It has been suggested that dyspepsia can be subdivided based on groups (or clusters) of symptoms. However, subgroups have not proved to be of value in identifying the underlying cause of dyspepsia and overlap considerably. Some patients report having troublesome burping associated with abdominal bloating or discomfort that is transiently relieved by bringing up the wind. These patients have aerophagy, and repeated swallowing of air may be obvious during the consultation.

Causes of dyspepsia

History taking is key to identifying the likely cause of dyspepsia.

Gastro-oesophageal reflux disease
It is important and practical to distinguish gastro-oesophageal reflux disease (GORD) from dyspepsia. Frequent heartburn is a cardinal symptom of GORD; acid reflux causes a retrosternal or epigastric burning feeling that characteristically radiates up towards the throat, is relieved transiently by antacids, and is precipitated by a meal or by lying down.

Up to 60% of people with upper gastrointestinal symptoms report both heartburn and epigastric pain or discomfort. This overlap can be confusing, but it is not the presence of a symptom but its predominance that is most helpful clinically. For example, if the main complaint is a burning epigastric pain that radiates up towards the throat then this is highly predictive of GORD (as can be objectively demonstrated by abnormal results from 24 hour oesophageal pH monitoring).

Reflux oesophagitis can be detected at endoscopy, but over half of patients with true GORD will not have evidence of mucosal breaks (erosions). Oesophageal erythema or the presence of a hiatal hernia are unreliable signs that cannot be used to determine if a patient has reflux disease. Although some patients are unable to adequately describe their symptoms or decide which is their predominant complaint, if a detailed history is taken a clinical diagnosis of GORD can be made in most cases, including those in whom endoscopy is normal.

Peptic ulcers
Many textbooks continue to propagate the myth that symptoms can accurately identify peptic ulcer disease. Unfortunately, classic ulcer symptoms (such as postprandial epigastric pain or night pain) often occur in patients with functional dyspepsia, and many patients with an ulcer have atypical complaints.

Box 10.1 Major structural causes of dyspepsia

- Chronic peptic ulcer (duodenal or gastric)
- Gastro-oesophageal reflux disease (>50% have no oesophagitis)
- Gastric or oesophageal adenocarcinoma (rare but of concern for patient and doctor)

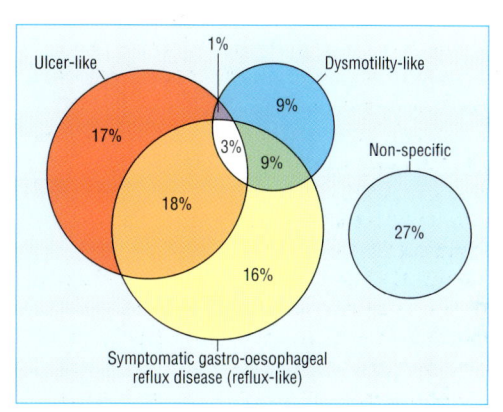

Figure 10.1 Overlap of subgroups of dyspepsia based on symptoms in patients with documented functional dyspepsia

---

Box 10.2 Uncommon causes of upper abdominal pain or discomfort that may be confused with dyspepsia

- Aerophagy (repetitive belching from air swallowing)
- Biliary colic from gall stones
- Abdominal wall pain (a clinical clue is localised tenderness on palpation not reduced by tensing the abdominal wall muscles)
- Chronic pancreatitis (episodic dull steady upper abdominal pain that may be aggravated by meals and radiate through to the back)
- Malignancy (such as of pancreas or colon)
- Mesenteric vascular insufficiency (postprandial pain, weight loss, and a fear of eating)
- Angina
- Metabolic disease (such as diabetes, renal failure, hypercalcaemia)

Box 10.3 Conditions to be recognised from a patient's history

Symptomatic gastro-ocsophageal reflux disease
- Burning retrosternal or epigastric pain or discomfort radiating upwards towards the throat and relieved, albeit transiently, by antacids
- Regurgitation of acid

Irritable bowel syndrome
- Abdominal pain plus an erratic disturbance of defecation linked to the pain (such as pain relief with defecation, looser or harder stools with pain onset, or more frequent or less frequent stools with pain onset)

Biliary tract disease
- Biliary-type pain

Peptic ulcer
- Classic ulcer symptoms do not distinguish peptic ulcer disease from functional dyspepsia

ABC of the Upper Gastrointestinal Tract

Endoscopy remains the test of choice to rule out chronic peptic ulceration, but its presence can now be inferred by indirect testing. *Helicobacter pylori* causes 90% of duodenal ulcers and 70% of gastric ulcers; aspirin and non-steroidal anti-inflammatory drugs (NSAIDs) account for most of the remainder. Patients who are not infected with *H pylori* and not taking NSAIDs have a very low probability of ulcer disease.

Gastric cancer
Fear of gastric cancer is one of the main reasons why patients with dyspepsia present to their general practitioner. Gastric cancer is found in less than 2% of all cases referred for endoscopy. Early gastric cancer comprises only 10% of cancer cases, but it is important to diagnose because it is curable and 60-90% of patients initially present with dyspepsia.

However, the risk of gastric cancer is extremely low in patients under the age of 55 years presenting with the new onset of dyspepsia in most Western countries including Britain. Furthermore, "alarm" symptoms such as weight loss, dysphagia, or anaemia help to identify those who need to be investigated in order to exclude malignancy, although between 15% and 50% of dyspeptic patients with gastric cancer do not have these symptoms. Endoscopic evaluation is therefore recommended in older patients presenting with new symptoms and in all patients with alarm symptoms.

Gall stones
Ultrasonography will detect gall stones in a minority of patients with apparently unexplained dyspepsia. However, gall stones are common and often incidental in the absence of biliary symptoms. Biliary colic is characteristically severe, episodic, and constant (rather than colicky) pain in the epigastrium or right upper quadrant typically lasting one to several hours. This can usually be easily distinguished from the pain or discomfort of functional dyspepsia.

While many patients with gall stones also complain of bloating, nausea, and other vague upper abdominal symptoms, these complaints are just as common in patients without gall stones. Moreover, cholecystectomy does not reliably result in long term relief of any of these vague complaints and cannot be recommended. Cholecystectomy in a patient with non-biliary type pain is likely to result in the patient at a later date being labelled as having the post-cholecystectomy syndrome.

Functional dyspepsia
Most commonly, either no abnormalities or irrelevant abnormalities (such as gastric erythema or a few gastric erosions) are found at endoscopy; these patients are labelled as having functional (or non-ulcer) dyspepsia. As antisecretory drugs may result in healing of ulcers or oesophagitis (and hence lead to a misdiagnosis of functional dyspepsia), these drugs are best not started before endoscopy if possible.

Functional dyspepsia

Pathogenesis
The pathogenesis of functional dyspepsia remains uncertain. *H pylori* gastritis is detected in about half of patients with functional dyspepsia, but it is also common in otherwise asymptomatic people. The question of whether this infection causes symptoms in patients without ulcer disease has been controversial. There is no evidence that specific symptoms identify those with *H pylori* infection. Acid secretion is usually normal in patients with functional dyspepsia, except perhaps in a subset infected with *H pylori*.

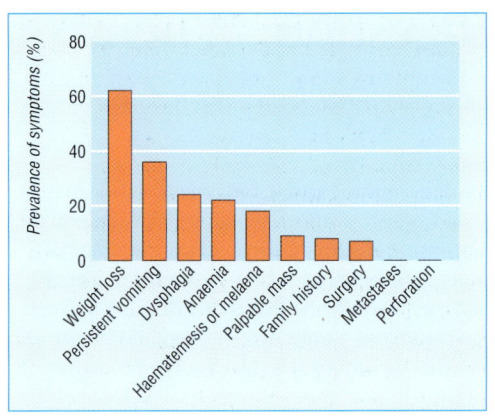

Figure 10.2 Prevalence of "alarm" symptoms in patients with gastric cancer

Box 10.4 Alarm symptoms
- Anorexia
- Loss of weight
- Anaemia due to iron deficiency
- Recent onset of persistent symptoms
- Melaena, haematemesis
- Dysphagia

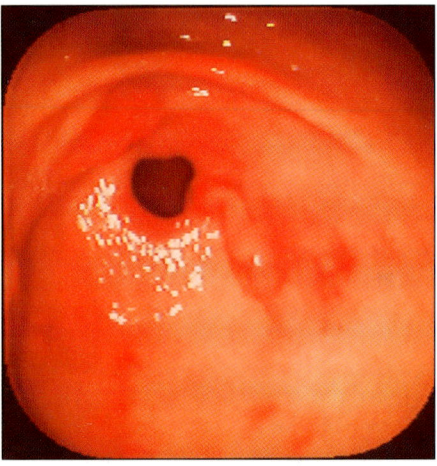

Figure 10.3 Antral erythema and erosions in patient with functional dyspepsia

Practice point
If possible, H_2 receptor antagonists and proton pump inhibitors should not be started before endoscopy (or should be stopped at least two weeks before endoscopy)

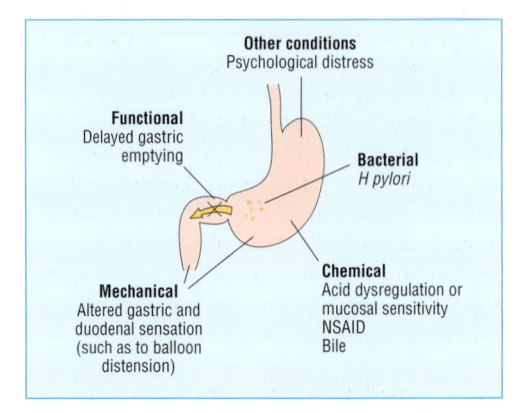

Figure 10.4 Pathogenesis of functional dyspepsia

Indigestion: When is it functional?

In functional dyspepsia gastric (and duodenal) sensation is disturbed (the "irritable stomach"), and in about half of patients distension induces symptoms at lower pressures or volumes than it does in healthy people. Delayed gastric emptying can be detected in a quarter to a half of patients with functional dyspepsia. In addition, a subset of patients have altered intragastric distribution of food, which reflects abnormal proximal gastric relaxation (a "stiff" fundus). There is an increased probability of detecting gastric motor abnormalities in women and possibly in those with severe postprandial fullness or severe vomiting.

There is controversy as to whether functional dyspepsia is a "forme fruste" of the irritable bowel syndrome, and both conditions may overlap. About a third of patients with functional dyspepsia have an erratic disturbance of defecation closely linked to their pain, and probably truly have irritable bowel syndrome. There is also evidence of gut hypersensitivity in both functional dyspepsia and the irritable bowel syndrome.

Smoking and alcohol do not seem to be important in functional dyspepsia, but coffee ingestion has been linked to exacerbation of symptoms. Some patients with functional dyspepsia suffer from an anxiety disorder or depression, but whether this is cause or effect remains unclear.

Identification and management

Investigation versus testing for H pylori
The devil is in the detail, and a careful detailed appraisal of a patient's history with a judicious approach to testing is necessary. Older patients or those with alarm features warrant prompt referral for endoscopy and further investigations as required. Testing for *H pylori* infection will help in guiding management in the remainder; between 20% and 60% of those with *H pylori* infection will have peptic ulcer disease.

For patients with *H pylori* infection, one course of action is to refer them for endoscopy to determine who has peptic ulcer disease or functional dyspepsia (the two main considerations) and plan treatment accordingly (the "test and endoscope" strategy). Alternatively, a reasonable course of action is to treat infected patients with appropriate antibiotics and observe the clinical course (the "test and treat" strategy). Although treatment of infection may not cure functional dyspepsia (see below), it will usually eliminate the peptic ulcer diathesis and hence will often relieve the symptoms. Moreover, recent trials suggest that "test and treat" is a safe and cost effective strategy that results in a long term outcome similar to that with a strategy of prompt endoscopy. Hence, "test and treat" has been gaining widespread acceptance.

Principles of management
Reassurance and explanation remain the key elements in managing documented or suspected functional dyspepsia. Patients should be advised that this is a real condition and that their symptoms are not imaginary. Furthermore, they should be advised that the condition never leads to cancer or other serious disease. Patients' fears should be identified and addressed. Modification of diet (such as avoiding foods that provoke symptoms and adopting a low fat diet because high fat foods may impair gastric emptying) and stopping medications can be helpful. Antacids are no better than placebo in functional dyspepsia, but notably the placebo response ranges between 20% and 60%.

Initial treatment
In patients with a diagnosis of functional dyspepsia, a short term therapeutic trial for four weeks with an acid suppressant is

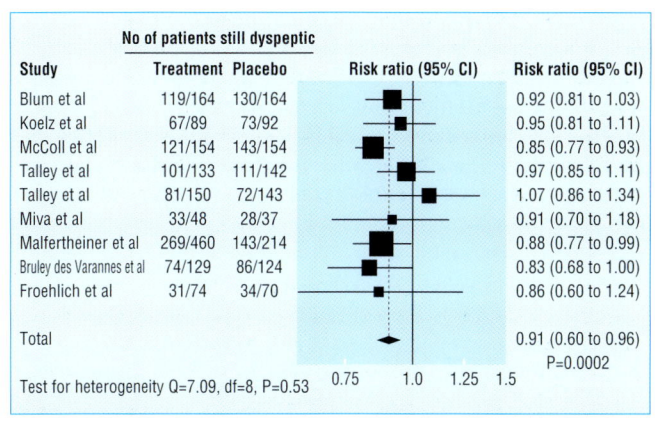

Study	Treatment	Placebo	Risk ratio (95% CI)
Blum et al	119/164	130/164	0.92 (0.81 to 1.03)
Koelz et al	67/89	73/92	0.95 (0.81 to 1.11)
McColl et al	121/154	143/154	0.85 (0.77 to 0.93)
Talley et al	101/133	111/142	0.97 (0.85 to 1.11)
Talley et al	81/150	72/143	1.07 (0.86 to 1.34)
Miva et al	33/48	28/37	0.91 (0.70 to 1.18)
Malfertheiner et al	269/460	143/214	0.88 (0.77 to 0.99)
Bruley des Varannes et al	74/129	86/124	0.83 (0.68 to 1.00)
Froehlich et al	31/74	34/70	0.86 (0.60 to 1.24)
Total			0.91 (0.60 to 0.96) P=0.0002

Test for heterogeneity Q=7.09, df=8, P=0.53

Figure 10.5 Results of systematic review comparing *H pylori* eradication treatment for non-ulcer dyspepsia with placebo

---

Box 10.5 Initial management of functional dyspepsia

- Make a positive clinical diagnosis
- Minimise investigations and don't repeat tests without good reason
- Determine the patient's agenda and identify psychosocial stressors
- Find out why the patient has presented now
- Provide education and reassurance

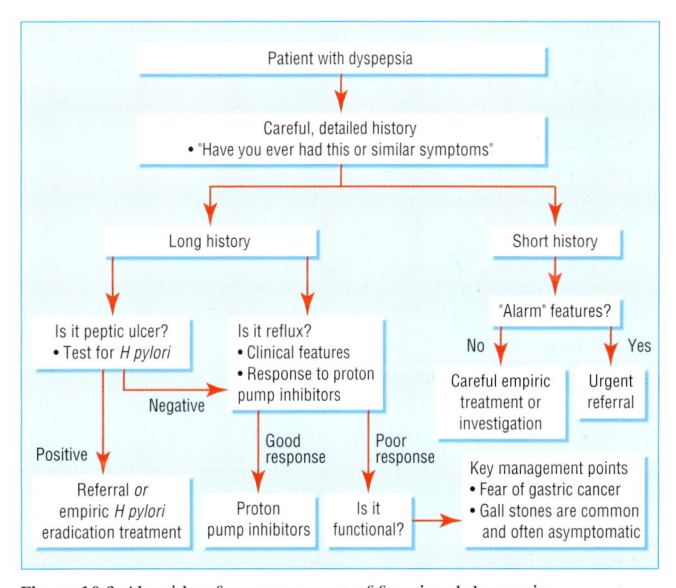

Figure 10.6 Algorithm for management of functional dyspepsia

Box 10.6 Drugs that are most likely to cause dyspepsia

- Non-steroidal anti-inflammatory drugs
- Digoxin
- Antibiotics (macrolides, metronidazole)
- Corticosteroids, oestrogens
- Iron, potassium chloride
- Levodopa
- Theophylline
- Quinidine
- Niacin, gemfibrozil
- Colchicine

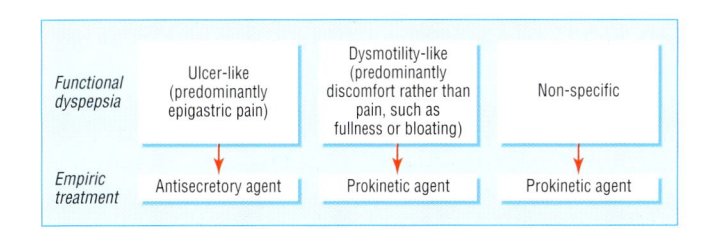

Figure 10.7 Empiric treatment for functional dyspepsia

Functional dyspepsia:
- Ulcer-like (predominantly epigastric pain) → Antisecretory agent
- Dysmotility-like (predominantly discomfort rather than pain, such as fullness or bloating) → Prokinetic agent
- Non-specific → Prokinetic agent

ABC of the Upper Gastrointestinal Tract

worth while. Symptom subgroups may be of some help in predicting a patient's response to treatment if a predominant symptom can be identified, but relying on clusters of symptoms is generally not useful.

H_2 receptor blockers are, at best, of only modest efficacy in functional dyspepsia. While some trials suggest that they are superior to placebo, other trials have not shown any additional benefit. Proton pump inhibitors are more efficacious than placebo in functional dyspepsia (by about 10-20%), but not in the subgroup of patients with dysmotility-like dyspepsia.

If a patient fails to respond to an antisecretory drug after four weeks, it is reasonable to consider increasing the dose or switching to an alternative or a prokinetic drug. If the patient has failed to respond after eight weeks, then it is reasonable to refer the case to a specialist for further evaluation.

Eradicating *H pylori* infection cures functional dyspepsia in only a minority of cases. A meta-analysis has suggested a small therapeutic gain over 12 months follow up (15 needed to be treated to cure one case). Whether sucralfate or bismuth is better than placebo in treating functional dyspepsia is unclear, but it is unlikely; misoprostol may actually aggravate symptoms and cause diarrhoea in some patients.

Long term management
Functional dyspepsia is generally a relapsing and remitting condition. Treatment should not be prolonged, and frequent drug holidays should be prescribed. In patients with symptoms that are difficult to control a trial of an antispasmodic or antidepressant may be useful, but specialist referral to confirm the diagnosis and exclude rare causes of dyspepsia should first be considered. Some patients will benefit from behavioural therapy or psychotherapy.

Aerophagy
Air swallowing is often extremely resistant to treatment. Options include avoidance of chewing gum, aerated drinks, and smoking; use of anti-gas agents (such as activated dimeticone or charcoal); and relaxation therapy. However, no treatment is of proved benefit, and anti-gas agents are no better than placebo.

The graph of prevalence of alarm symptoms in patients with gastric cancer is adapted from Gillen D, McColl KE. *Am J Gastroenterol* 1999;94:75-9. The forest plot comparing *H pylori* eradication treatment with placebo is reproduced from Moayyedi P, et al. *BMJ* 2000;321:659-64.

Box 10.7 Treatment for functional dyspepsia
Initial treatment
- Antisecretory drug (H_2 receptor blocker, proton pump inhibitor)
or
- Prokinetic drug (domperidone) if antisecretory treatment fails
- Switch treatment if first drug type fails

Resistant cases (failed initial treatment)
- *H pylori* eradication
- Sucralfate or bismuth
- Antispasmodic agent (such as mebeverine)
- Antidepressant (such as selective serotonin reuptake inhibitor or tricyclic drug)
- Behavioural therapy or psychotherapy
- No treatment is proved to be of benefit in these patients

Box 10.8 When to consider referring a dyspeptic patient to a specialist
- If prompt investigation is required (such as recent onset of alarm symptoms)
- Severe pain
- Failure of symptoms to resolve or substantially improve after appropriate treatment
- Progressive symptoms

11 Upper abdominal pain: Gall bladder

C D Johnson

Gall stones are common but often do not give rise to symptoms. Pain arising from the gall bladder may be typical of biliary colic, but a wide variety of atypical presentations can make the diagnosis challenging. After a period of uncertainty in the 1980s, when operative techniques were challenged by drug treatment and lithotripsy, it is now widely accepted that symptomatic gallbladder stones should be treated by laparoscopic cholecystectomy. Clinical judgment and local expertise will greatly influence the management of bile duct stones, particularly if cholecystectomy is also required.

> **Asymptomatic gall stones are common and require no treatment**
> **Typical symptoms include biliary colic—right upper quadrant pain, radiating to the back, and lasting less than 12 hours**
> **Symptomatic gall stones are usually treated by laparoscopic cholecystectomy**

Epidemiology of gall stones

In the United Kingdom about 8% of the population aged over 40 years have gall stones, which rises to over 20% in those aged over 60. Fortunately, 90% of these stones remain asymptomatic, but cholecystectomy is the most commonly performed abdominal procedure.

The incidence of gall stones varies widely, being greatly influenced by dietary intake, particularly of fat. For example, in Saudi Arabia gallstone disease was virtually unheard of 50 years ago, but, with increasing affluence and a Western type diet, gall stones are now as common there as in many Western countries. Genetic factors also contribute. The native Indian populations of Chile and Peru are highly susceptible, with a close to 100% lifetime risk of gall stones in their female population. Several risk factors have been identified, which relate to the two major stone types, cholesterol stones and pigment stones.

Pathogenesis

Gall stones form when the solubility of bilirubin or cholesterol is exceeded. Pigment stones arise in the gall bladder when there has been increased bilirubin production from breakdown of haemoglobin. Mixed stones contain both bilirubin and cholesterol and may be calcified. Precipitated bilirubin may form a nidus for subsequent cholesterol deposition.

Secondary pigment stones form in the bile duct as a consequence of obstruction or by accumulation around a small primary stone. These stones are associated with bacterial infection and arise by bacterial deconjugation of the bilirubin-glucuronide complex.

Cholesterol stones arise because of an imbalance in the mechanisms maintaining cholesterol in solution. Cholesterol is a hydrophobic molecule and is dispersed in micelles by the combined action of bile salts and lecithin. The risk of precipitation is directly related to cholesterol concentration and inversely to the concentrations of bile salts and lecithin, giving rise to a triangular coordinate. Increased cholesterol excretion is largely of dietary origin but may also result from changes in steroid metabolism associated with pregnancy, oral contraceptives, and obesity.

Bile salts are retrieved from the gut by the terminal ileum, and this enterohepatic circulation is essential for maintenance of the bile salt pool. The endogenous synthesis of bile salt is rate limited at a level much lower than its normal daily excretion by the liver. Many gastrointestinal diseases affect bile salt metabolism—in particular, Crohn's disease and surgical resection of the terminal ileum predispose people to gall stones.

Box 11.1 Risk factors for gall stones

Cholesterol stones
- Obesity
- High fat diet
- Oestrogens (female, pregnancy, oral contraception)
- Hereditary
- Loss of bile salts (Crohn's disease, terminal ileal resection)
- Impaired gall bladder emptying (such as truncal vagotomy, type 1 diabetes, octreotide, parenteral nutrition, and starvation or rapid voluntary weight loss)

Pigment stones
- Haemolytic disease
- Biliary stasis
- Biliary infection

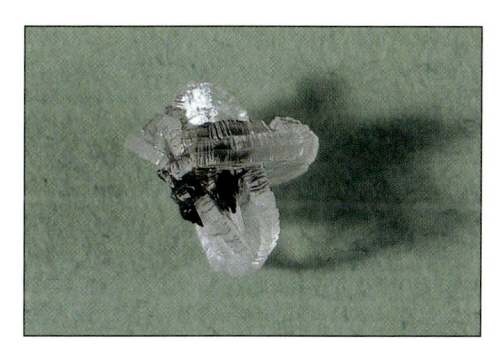

Figure 11.1 Mixed gall stone with bilirubin nucleus and attached clear cholesterol crystals

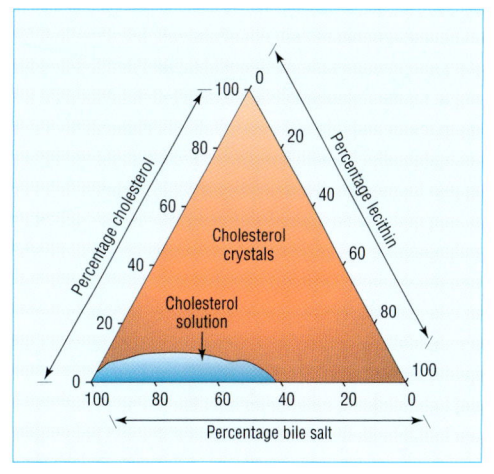

Figure 11.2 Triangular coordinates relating solubility of cholesterol with concentrations of cholesterol, bile salts, and lecithin

ABC of the Upper Gastrointestinal Tract

Impaired gallbladder emptying predisposes to gall stones by increasing the time that material stays in the gall bladder, allowing excessive crystal growth. In addition, the dilating and flushing effect of fresh hepatic bile is lost when the gall bladder contracts poorly.

Symptoms associated with gall stones

Biliary colic is usually felt as a severe gripping or gnawing pain in the right upper quadrant. It may radiate to the epigastrium, or around the lower ribs, or directly through to the back. It may be referred to the lower pole of the scapula or the right lower ribs posteriorly. However, many variations on this pattern have been described, including retrosternal pain and abdominal pain only in the epigastrium or on the left side. Such symptoms, in the presence of gallbladder stones, merit consideration of cholecystectomy.

There may be difficulty when symptoms are less clear. In a year about 25% of the adult population consults a general practitioner for dyspeptic symptoms. As nearly 8% of these individuals will have asymptomatic gall stones, many patients with dyspeptic symptoms are given the label "gallstone dyspepsia." A pattern of symptoms supposedly associated with gall stones has been described, but several careful studies of patients before and after cholecystectomy have failed to show any clear association with either a good or poor outcome. Since asymptomatic gall stones and dyspepsia are so common in the general populations, they often coexist. Dyspeptic symptoms may be too readily attributed to the presence of gall stones, leading to inappropriate and ineffective surgery. Not surprisingly, therefore, symptoms may persist in up to 20% of patients after cholecystectomy.

Complications

Gallbladder stones may be complicated by acute cholecystitis, mucocele, or empyema. These are difficult to distinguish clinically; a patient may present with an episode of acute cholecystitis that fails to resolve and at operation is found to have an empyema or a mucocele. In addition to symptoms of biliary colic, such patients have pain that is constant and lasts for more than 12 hours; they also have tenderness over the gall bladder, which may be palpable, and may have a fever and leucocytosis.

Complications of bile duct stones include obstructive jaundice and acute pancreatitis.

Any patient with suspected complications of either gallbladder or bile duct stones should be referred for urgent specialist assessment and may well require immediate admission to hospital.

Diagnosis

Ultrasonography has replaced cholecystography as the diagnostic test for gall stones. About 95% of gallbladder stones will be detected by ultrasonography, which is cheap, quick, and harmless. If strong clinical suspicion of gall stones exist, and ultrasonography does not show stones, the test should be repeated. Other diagnostic tests are less sensitive and are rarely indicated.

Management

The management of gall stones depends on their position, either in the gall bladder or bile duct.

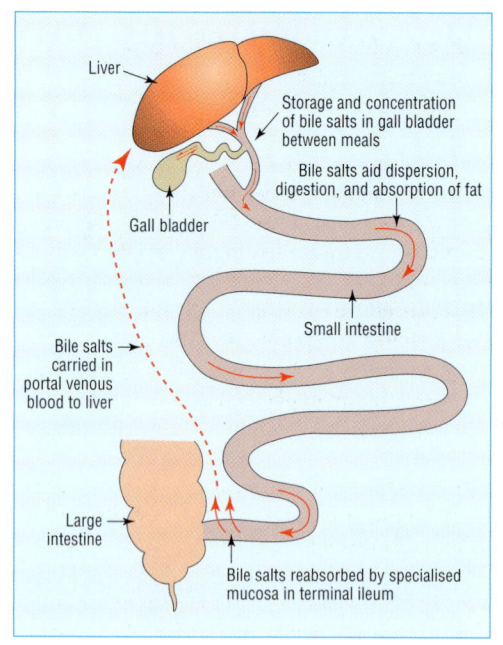

Figure 11.3 Enterohepatic circulation of bile salts. Each molecule circulates at least once for each meal

---

Box 11.2 Symptoms associated with gall stones

Biliary colic
- Right subcostal or epigastric pain radiating to back or lower pole of scapula lasting for 20 minutes to 6 hours
- Associated with vomiting brought on by (any) food
- May disturb sleep

Acute cholecystitis
- Severe pain and tenderness in right subcostal region for >12 hours
- Fever and leucocytosis

Obstructive jaundice with or without pain

Box 11.3 Symptoms of dyspepsia *not* associated with gall stones

- Repeated belching
- Inability to finish normal meals
- Fluid regurgitation
- Nausea
- Fullness after normal meals
- Abdominal distension (bloating)
- Epigastric or retrosternal burning
- Vomiting (without biliary colic)

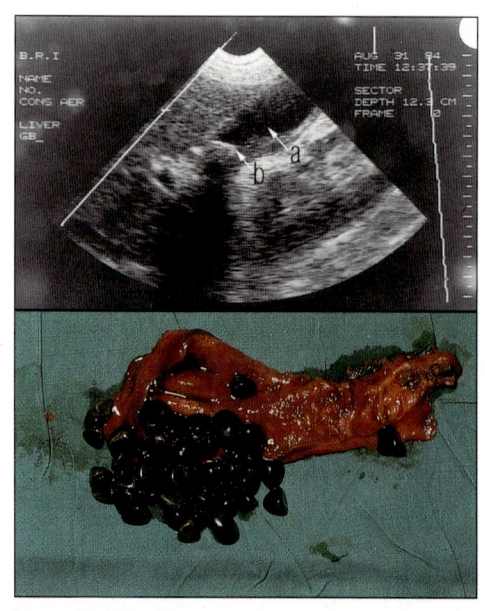

Figure 11.4 Top: Ultrasound image of gall bladder with dark area (a) representing gall bladder and multiple white echoes (b) representing stones. Bottom: The gall bladder after cholecystectomy with multiple small stones

Upper abdominal pain: Gall bladder

Gallbladder stones

The management of gallbladder stones is now relatively straightforward. Asymptomatic gallstones require no intervention as the risks of any procedure outweigh the potential benefits.

In the 1980s dissatisfaction with the outcome of open cholecystectomy led to several alternative therapies such as extracorporeal shock wave lithotripsy and bile salt dissolution therapy. These treatments were restricted in their applicability and have been almost completely superseded by laparoscopic cholecystectomy. This procedure offers a more rapid recovery and return to work, much less abdominal scarring, and at least as good long term relief of symptoms as open cholecystectomy. In specialist hands almost all uncomplicated gallbladder stones can be dealt with laparoscopically, with minimal risk of injury to the bile duct.

Complicated gallbladder stones—If complications arise (such as acute cholecystitis, mucocele, or empyema) cholecystectomy is performed. This will usually be by the laparoscopic approach, but up to 10% of operations have to be converted to laparotomy. In some elderly patients with acute presentation, percutaneous cholecystostomy is performed under ultrasound control to relieve the infection and avoid the morbidity of an emergency operation. Subsequently, the stones may be extracted percutaneously, leaving the gall bladder in place, or, if appropriate, cholecystectomy is performed.

Stones in the bile duct

Stones may migrate from the gall bladder into the bile duct. Cholangiography is performed before, during, or immediately after cholecystectomy to demonstrate the presence or absence of bile duct stones in patients with known risk factors. A cholangiogram may be obtained endoscopically, at operation, or by means of magnetic resonance imaging. Uncomplicated bile duct stones should be removed when they are detected, because of the high risk of complications such as acute pancreatitis, obstructive jaundice, or cholangitis if they are left in situ.

The management of asymptomatic duct stones is controversial. The traditional approach of open cholecystectomy with exploration of the common bile duct offers simplicity and widespread applicability and avoids exposing the patient to the risk of procedure related pancreatitis. Alternatives are laparoscopic cholecystectomy with endoscopic sphincterotomy and stone extraction either before or after cholecystectomy, or else laparoscopic exploration of the common bile duct. Currently practice varies according to the expertise available locally.

Acalculous biliary pain

The symptoms of biliary colic are characteristic but may occur in the absence of gall stones. In such cases a specialist must decide whether an operation to remove the gall bladder is appropriate, in the belief that symptoms are due to microscopic crystals (microlithiasis) or to a structural abnormality of the cystic duct.

Occasionally, biliary colic seems to be associated with a high pressure sphincter of Oddi, and symptoms may resolve after endoscopic sphincterotomy. Alternative explanations for so called acalculous biliary pain include irritable bowel syndrome with upper gastrointestinal manifestations (see previous article). Chronic pancreatitis must also be carefully excluded. Any decision to carry out a cholecystectomy for this condition should be made by a hepatobiliary specialist.

Box 11.4 Options for treatment of symptomatic gallbladder disease

Laparoscopic cholecystectomy—Safe in specialist hands, rapid recovery, permanently effective, current gold standard
Open cholecystectomy—Traditional, painful, prolonged recovery, scar

Alternative therapies

Extracorporeal shock wave lithotripsy—Complex
Bile salt dissolution—Expensive
Percutaneous cholecyslithotomy—Leaves abnormal gall bladder in situ, high recurrence rate, suitable only for a few selected patients

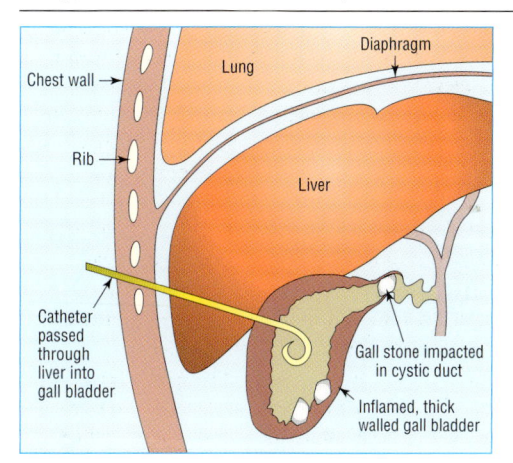

Figure 11.5 Percutaneous cholecystostomy for acute cholecystitis. Percutaneous drainage relieves the acute phase, allowing subsequent stone extraction via the drain track or cholecystectomy when inflammation has resolved

---

Box 11.5 Risk factors suggesting presence of bile duct stones at cholecystectomy for symptomatic gallbladder stones

- Common bile duct dilated (>6 mm on ultrasound)
- Recent abnormal levels of liver enzymes or bilirubin
- History of acute pancreatitis
- History of obstructive jaundice

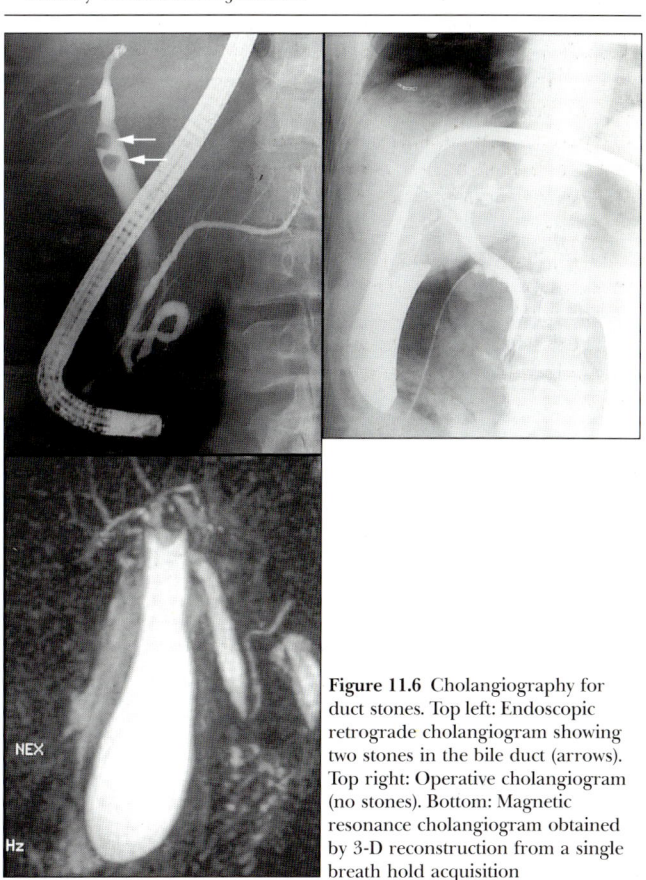

Figure 11.6 Cholangiography for duct stones. Top left: Endoscopic retrograde cholangiogram showing two stones in the bile duct (arrows). Top right: Operative cholangiogram (no stones). Bottom: Magnetic resonance cholangiogram obtained by 3-D reconstruction from a single breath hold acquisition

Gallbladder cancer

Gallbladder cancer is rare and usually asymptomatic until at an advanced stage. Usually it is associated with gall stones and may be discovered incidentally at operation. Suspicious features in a patient with biliary symptoms include weight loss, anaemia, persistent vomiting, and a palpable mass in the right upper quadrant. Such patients require urgent investigation. The prognosis is good if the disease is diagnosed at an early stage, but complete resection is often not possible because of the advanced stage at presentation.

The diagram of triangular coordinates relating cholesterol solubility with bile salts and lecithin is adapted from Admirand WH, Small DM. *J Clin Invest* 1968;47:1043-52. The magnetic resonance cholangiogram was kindly provided by Dr C N Hacking.

12 Cancer of the stomach and pancreas

Matthew J Bowles, Irving S Benjamin

Cancers of the stomach and the pancreas share similarly poor prognoses. However, long term survival is possible if patients present at an early stage. In England and Wales carcinoma of the stomach and pancreas cause about 7% and 4% of all cancer deaths respectively. In women they are the fourth and fifth most common causes of cancer death; in men their respective rankings are third equal (with colonic cancer) and seventh.

The incidence of distal gastric carcinoma has fallen in the West, probably because of decreasing rates of infection with *Helicobacter pylori*, but it remains one of the main causes of death from malignancy worldwide. The incidence of proximal gastric cancer seems to be rising. These two gastric cancers depend on the distribution and severity of *H pylori* gastritis, as discussed in the earlier chapter on the pathophysiology of duodenal and gastric ulcers and gastric cancer.[1]

Cancer of the stomach

Gastric adenocarcinoma is rare below the age of 40 years, and its incidence peaks at about 60 years of age. Men are affected twice as often as women. Chronic atrophic pangastritis associated with *H pylori* infection is one of the most important risk factors for distal gastric cancer.

Clinical presentation

Symptoms may not occur until local disease is advanced. Patients may have symptoms and signs related to secondary spread (principally to the liver) and to the general effects of advanced malignancy, such as weight loss, anorexia, or nausea. Epigastric pain is present in about 80% of patients and may be similar to that from a benign gastric ulcer. If caused by obstruction of the gastric lumen, it is relieved by vomiting. Carcinoma of the gastric cardia may cause dysphagia.

Constant abdominal pain, and particularly back pain, are sinister symptoms implying local invasion by tumour. Chronic or acute bleeding from the tumour may occur, with consequent symptoms. There is often little to be found on examination, but there may be a palpable epigastric mass. The classic Troisier's sign (left supraclavicular lymph node enlargement) is rare.

Investigations and staging

Endoscopy and barium meal are the principal investigations. Endoscopy allows direct visualisation and biopsy of the carcinoma. Differentiation between benign and malignant gastric ulcers at endoscopy can be difficult, and several biopsies are therefore taken (ideally six) from all parts of the ulcer. Diagnostic accuracy approaches 100% if 10 samples are taken. A benign gastric ulcer is probably not a premalignant condition.

A barium study gives a better impression of the anatomy of the tumour and the degree of obstruction. It is also helpful for diagnosis of linitis plastica, which may be missed at gastroscopy. In the presence of dysphagia it is important to request a barium swallow and meal rather than a barium meal alone.

Endoscopy and barium studies are complementary. If the first investigation is negative in a patient with sinister symptoms the other test is indicated. If a diagnosis of benign ulceration is made it is essential to repeat the endoscopy and biopsies after

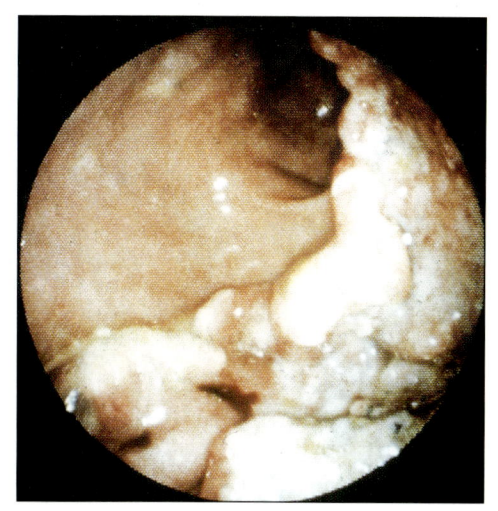

Figure 12.1 Endoscopic appearance of gastric carcinoma on the lesser curve of the stomach

---

Box 12.1 Risk factors for gastric cancer

- *H pylori* infection and atrophic gastritis
- Pernicious anaemia
- Adenomatous gastric polyps
- Partial gastrectomy
- Abnormalities in E-cadherin gene
- Family history of gastric cancer

Box 12.2 Signs and symptoms of gastric cancer

Symptoms	Signs

• Pain
  Epigastric
  Back (advanced)
• Anorexia
• Vomiting
• Dysphagia
• Iron deficiency anaemia
• Haematemesis or melaena
• Weight loss
	• Cachexia, weight loss, anaemia
	• Epigastric mass
	• Hepatomegaly
	• Palpable left supraclavicular node (Troisier's sign)

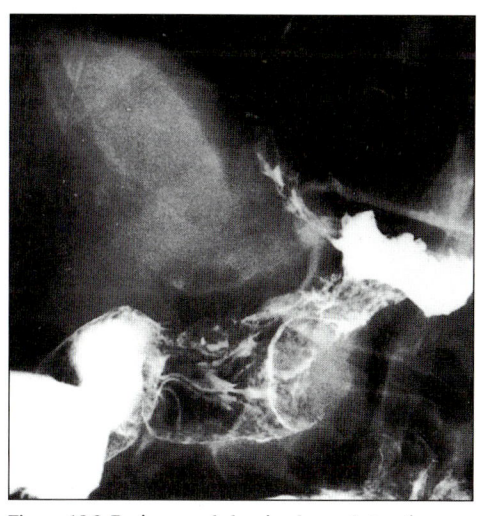

Figure 12.2 Barium meal showing large obstructing carcinoma of the body of the stomach

ABC of the Upper Gastrointestinal Tract

four to eight weeks of medical treatment to confirm ulcer healing and the benign nature of the lesion.

Staging of the disease by computed tomography of the thorax and abdomen, and sometimes by laparoscopy or endoscopic ultrasonography, is appropriate only in those patients who are proceeding to surgery.

Differential diagnosis

Once a gastroscopy or barium study has been performed, there are usually few problems with the diagnosis of gastric carcinoma. The difficulty lies in deciding which patients need urgent investigation of their presenting symptoms. A good initial symptomatic response to acid suppression does not exclude malignancy. Guidelines from the British Society of Gastroenterology for the investigation of dyspepsia suggest that all patients aged over 45 years should undergo endoscopy, whereas those under 45 need endoscopy only if they have symptoms or signs that raise suspicion of malignancy.

Treatment

Curative treatment

The decision to perform a gastrectomy depends on the patient's general state of health and nutrition and the preoperative staging of the cancer. If there is no evidence of local invasion or of metastatic spread, resection is offered as a potential cure. Overall perioperative mortality is about 2%. Long term survival depends principally on the extent of lymph node metastases.

Chemotherapy may have an increasingly important role to play in treating gastric carcinoma. Recent emphasis has been on preoperative chemotherapy in order to "downstage" the tumour. There seems to be little place for radiotherapy in the treatment of gastric carcinoma at present.

Palliative treatment

Patients with distal obstructing tumours may benefit from a subtotal gastrectomy or gastrojejunostomy despite the presence of metastases. Stenting of tumours of the gastric cardia relieves dysphagia. Other treatments include endoscopic laser therapy for unresectable obstruction or bleeding lesions. Blood transfusion may be appropriate for symptomatic anaemia. The management of pain from gastric carcinoma follows established palliative care practice. Coeliac plexus nerve blocks may be effective. As with any malignant condition, the management of symptoms is multidisciplinary and is often led by palliative care and hospice based teams.

Prognosis

The disease is incurable in about half of patients at presentation. With regional lymph node metastases, five year survival after gastrectomy is about 10%. In those with only perigastric lymph node involvement survival rises to 30%, and in those with gastric carcinoma confined to the stomach five year survival is about 70%. Only 10% of patients with hepatic metastases survive a year.

Early gastric cancer

Early gastric cancer is a carcinoma diagnosed before it has penetrated the full thickness of the stomach wall or metastasised, but this accounts for less than 5% of gastric carcinomata in the West. In Japan, where the incidence of gastric carcinoma is much higher (about 10%), population screening detects a far greater proportion of asymptomatic early gastric cancer. With aggressive surgery, five year survival rates of 90% have been reported from Japan. It is unclear, however, whether these differences in survival are due to early detection, differences in the disease or its pathological definition, or operative technique.

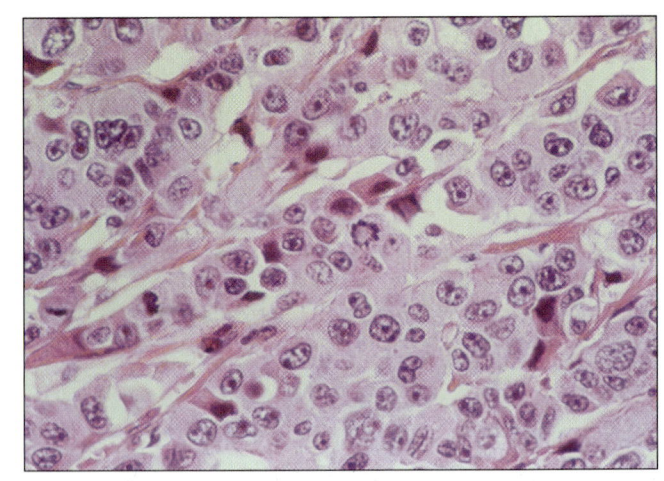

Figure 12.3 Light micrograph of human stomach cancer. Most of the cells seen here are cancerous, having large, irregular shapes and multiple nuclei

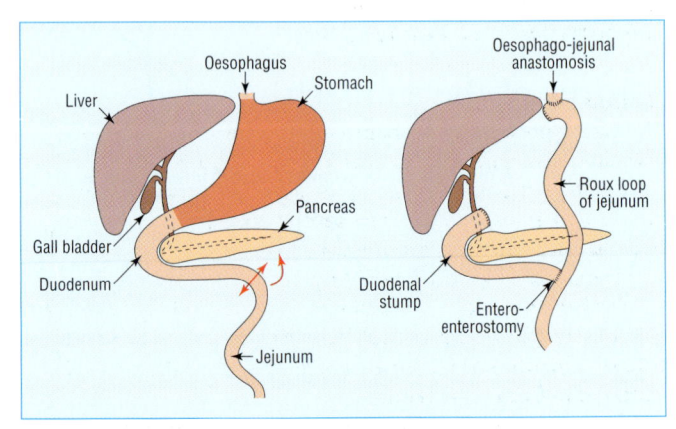

Figure 12.4 Total gastrectomy for treatment of gastric cancer (left) and subsequent reconstruction by Roux-en-Y anastomosis (right)

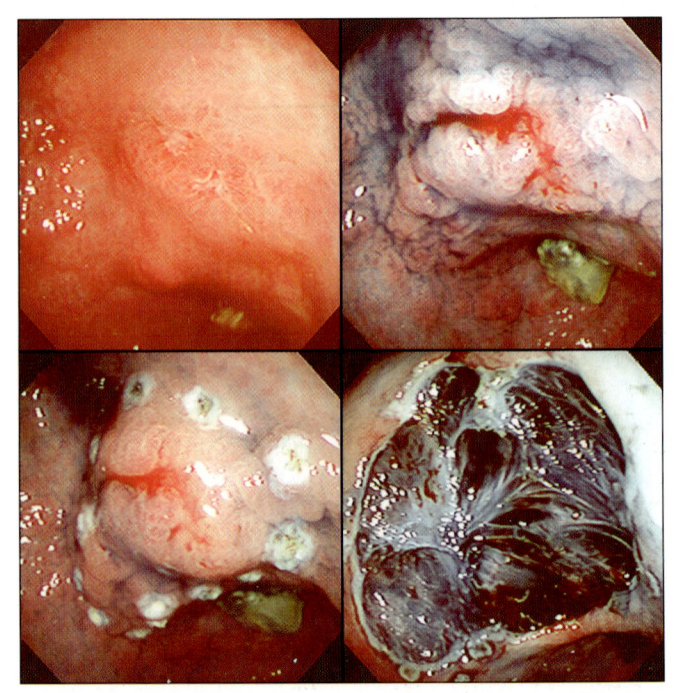

Figure 12.5 Early gastric cancer. Top left: endoscopic appearance of cancer before dye spraying. Top right: the same lesion after spraying with 0.2% indigo carmine dye. Bottom left: lesion outlined by burn marks before excision. Bottom right: mucosal defect after removal of the lesion with 1 cm margin (blue colour is due to indigo carmine dye)

Cancer of the pancreas

The incidence of pancreatic cancer is about 10 per 100 000 population in Western Europe. The incidence rises steadily with age, and the disease is slightly more common in men than in women. Alcohol, chronic pancreatitis, diabetes, and coffee do not predispose to pancreatic cancer.

Pathological features
The commonest pancreatic neoplasm is ductal adenocarcinoma. Most cancers arise in the head, neck, or uncinate process of the pancreas and may compress the common bile duct. Less than a third occur in the body and tail of the pancreas.

Periampullary malignancies may arise from the pancreas, the distal common bile duct, the ampulla of Vater, or the duodenum. Pancreatic carcinoma accounts for up to 90% of this group, but the rest are important—periampullary tumours present early because they obstruct the common bile duct and cause jaundice when they are small, so they have better prognoses than pancreatic carcinoma.

Clinical presentation
The classic presentation is painless, progressive, obstructive jaundice. Most patients also have epigastric discomfort or dull back pain. A large carcinoma of the head of the pancreas may obstruct the gastric outlet. Symptoms from a carcinoma of the body or tail of the pancreas are usually more vague, and the tumour is often locally advanced by the time of diagnosis.

Steatorrhoea may sometimes occur as a result of pancreatic duct obstruction and may be difficult to differentiate from the pale stool of obstructive jaundice. There are also the general effects of malignant disease.

The patient is usually jaundiced and may be anaemic or cachectic. There may be an epigastric mass or an irregular, enlarged liver because of metastases. Courvoisier's law states that, in the presence of jaundice, a palpable gall bladder is unlikely to be due to gall stones. This is because stones usually result in a fibrotic gall bladder, which will not distend in the presence of obstruction of the common bile duct.

Investigations and staging
Serum biochemistry will confirm jaundice and also give some information about its cause: alkaline phosphatase and γ-glutamyltransferase tend to be predominantly raised in obstructive jaundice. Disproportionate elevation of the aminotransferases (transaminases) leads to suspicion of hepatocellular involvement. Tumour markers may be of value in diagnosis: carcinoembryonic antigen (the marker associated with colonic carcinoma) is elevated in up to 85% of cases. Raised serum levels of CA 19.9 are associated with carcinoma of the pancreas but also with obstruction of the common bile duct from any cause. Lack of tumour markers should not delay investigation of jaundiced patients; their main use is in monitoring response to treatment and disease progression.

Ultrasonography is the initial investigation for patients with jaundice. A dilated common bile duct or intrahepatic ducts differentiate obstructive (posthepatic) jaundice from prehepatic and hepatic jaundice. Liver metastases are easily detected.

Endoscopic retrograde cholangiopancreatography visualises the common bile and pancreatic duct, and carcinoma of the head of the pancreas produces a characteristic malignant stricture of the lower end of the common bile duct. Brushings can be taken for cytological analysis, and the stricture may be dilated and stented to re-establish bile drainage into the

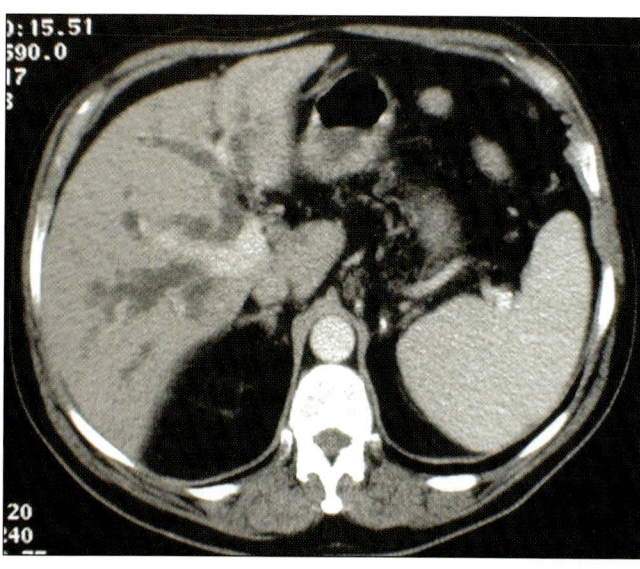

Figure 12.6 Computed tomogram showing dilated intrahepatic ducts caused by an obstructing lesion of the lower end of the common bile duct

---

Box 12.3 Risk factors for pancreatic cancer
- Smoking
- Partial gastrectomy
- Dietary fat
- Family history of pancreatic cancer

Box 12.4 Signs and symptoms of pancreatic cancer

Symptoms
- Obstructive jaundice—dark urine, pale stools, pruritus
- Pain
  Back (common)
  Epigastric
- Vomiting
- Weight loss
- Anorexia
- Haematemesis or melaena (late)

Signs
- Jaundice
- Cachexia, anaemia
- Epigastric mass (late)
- Palpable gall bladder (Courvoisier's sign)

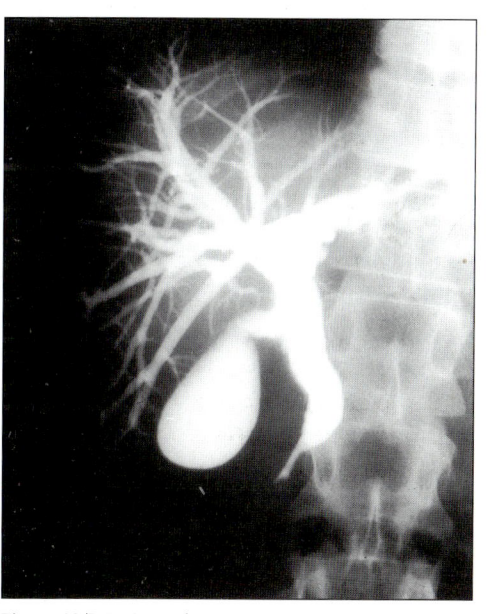

Figure 12.7 Endoscopic retrograde cholangiopancreatography showing lower common bile duct stricture (endoscope has been withdrawn)

ABC of the Upper Gastrointestinal Tract

duodenum. The main complication is acute pancreatitis, especially if therapeutic procedures are performed.

Computed tomography further assesses the primary tumour and detects lymph node involvement and hepatic or pulmonary metastases. If a mass is seen a fine needle aspirate can be taken under tomographic or ultrasound guidance for cytology, which has a sensitivity (a positive result when tumour is present) of about 70%. A core biopsy for histology can also be obtained.

Differential diagnosis

Anicteric patients with pancreatic carcinoma are usually initially investigated for their pain by gastroscopy or ultrasonography. Unless good views of the pancreas are obtained by the latter, computed tomography is required for the diagnosis.

Chronic pancreatitis may have a similar presentation, but there is usually a history of alcohol misuse. However, the two conditions may be radiologically indistinguishable, and fine needle aspiration cytology or histological assessment is needed. For prognosis, it is important to distinguish malignant periampullary lesions from tumours of the head of the pancreas.

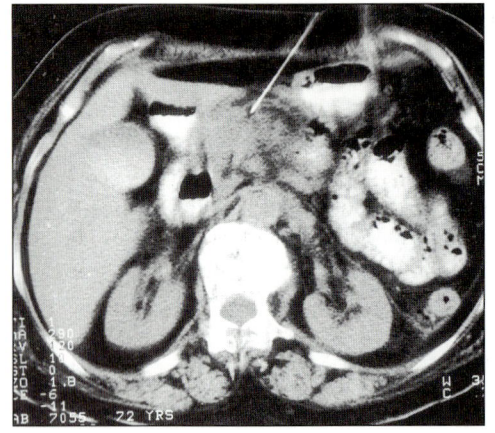

Figure 12.8 Fine needle aspiration of a pancreatic mass under computed tomographic guidance

Treatment

Surgery provides the only realistic hope of long term survival, but it is of value only if the primary tumour is no more than a few centimetres in diameter and is free of major blood vessels and if there is no metastatic spread. Unfortunately, few patients meet these criteria.

Suitable patients undergo Whipple's procedure. The head of the pancreas, the distal common bile duct, the gall bladder, and the duodenum and distal stomach are excised. Reconstruction involves anastomosis of the pancreatic duct, the common hepatic duct, and the distal stomach to a loop of jejunum. Perioperative mortality is now less than 5% in experienced hands, and complication rates have decreased, but Whipple's procedure remains a formidable operation, and patients must be fit in order to be suitable. A modification allows preservation of the distal stomach and pylorus, which may have long term nutritional benefits.

Distal pancreatectomy may be suitable for carcinoma of the body or tail, but few patients are suitable. Total pancreatectomy and extended vascular resections are rarely advocated.

Postoperative chemotherapy has been shown to be of some benefit after pancreatic resection, and there is currently much interest in the role of new chemotherapeutic agents in pancreatic cancer. Postoperative radiotherapy has proved ineffective.

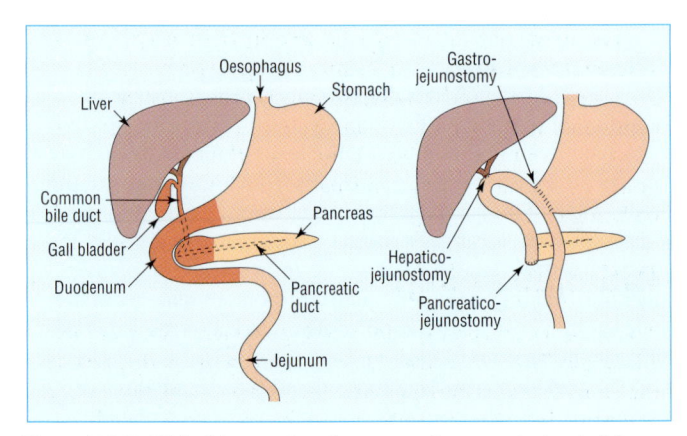

Figure 12.9 In Whipple's procedure for pancreatic cancer the head of the pancreas, distal common bile duct, gall bladder, duodenum, and distal stomach are excised (left). Reconstruction involves anastomosis of the pancreatic duct, common hepatic duct, and distal stomach to a loop of jejunum (right)

Palliative treatment

Jaundice is palliated by stenting the stricture at the lower end of the common bile duct; this has superseded operative palliation. Some 15-20% of patients develop duodenal obstruction, which can be relieved by laparoscopic gastrojejunostomy. There is no indication for prophylactic gastrojejunostomy, because most patients die of their disease before duodenal obstruction becomes a problem.

Palliation of pain and of other symptoms is best managed by a hospice based multidisciplinary palliative care team. Coeliac plexus block is often extremely valuable.

Prognosis

The prognosis of unresectable pancreatic carcinoma is poor, with few patients surviving longer than a year from diagnosis. Five year survival after resection for pancreatic carcinoma has steadily improved and is now 10-20% in major centres. This rises to about 50% for resection of periampullary tumours.

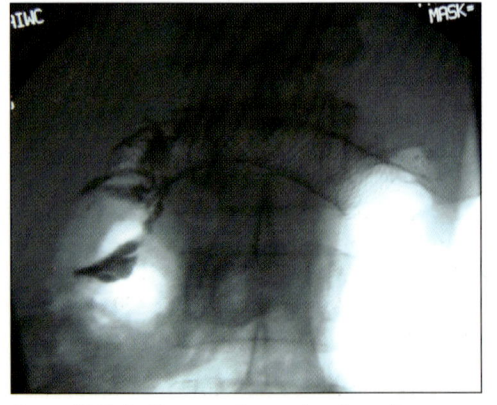

Figure 12.10 Radiogram of stent placed to relieve duodenal obstruction caused by carcinoma of the pancreas

1 Calam J, Baron JH. ABC of the upper gastrointestinal tract: Pathophysiology of duodenal and gastric ulcer and gastric cancer. *BMJ* 2001;323:980-2.

The light micrograph of gastric cancer cells is reproduced with permission of Science Photo Library/Parviz M Pour.

13 Anorexia, nausea, vomiting, and pain

R C Spiller

With the steady decline in diseases associated with *Helicobacter pylori* infection, the commonest diagnosis, both in general practice and hospital outpatients, is increasingly likely to be functional dyspepsia, a condition that is ill understood and for which management is poorly defined.

Prevalence of symptoms

Although upper abdominal and epigastric pain is extremely common and hence a poor discriminator of disease, only 2-8% of the general population experience anorexia, nausea, and vomiting, and so these are much more likely to indicate disease. Thankfully, many of these events turn out to be short lived, and only about 25% of those affected consult their general practitioner, but this still accounts for 1-2% of all consultations in general practice.

Two thirds of patients give the severity of their symptoms as a reason for consulting, but a similar proportion consult because of fear of serious disease, a factor that must be considered when planning management. The challenge is to reliably sift out and satisfactorily reassure the 40% with functional disease without missing those with more serious pathology.

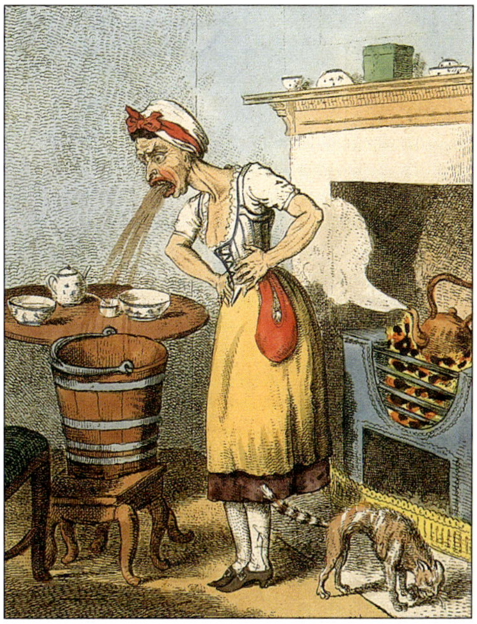

Pathophysiology

Anorexia, nausea, and vomiting with pain can all be regarded teleologically as protective reflexes whereby the body prevents the entry of toxins into the body. They also reduce the passage of chyme through diseased parts of the upper gut, thereby minimising further pain.

There are many possible organic causes, but, because there is an important central component, these behaviour patterns can be learnt and may be anticipatory. Thus, patients about to receive chemotherapy may vomit at the sight of the drugs, which they have previously associated with vomiting. Anxiety and depression can also be associated with alterations in taste—with associated anorexia, nausea, and weight loss—through neural pathways as yet poorly defined.

Pharmacology

Toxins and hypertonic saline induce vomiting by stimulating afferent serotonergic nerves in the vagus that connect with the chemoreceptive trigger zone in the floor of the fourth ventricle of the brain. These afferent nerves can also respond to acid, amino acids, and fatty acids. 5-HT$_3$ receptor antagonists act on the vagal afferents to reduce nausea and emesis. The chemoreceptive trigger zone also responds to bloodborne stimuli such as apomorphine, resulting in vomiting. Dopamine 2 receptor blockers act here to inhibit emesis and the subjective sense of nausea that precedes it. Excessive distension of the gut will induce pain via serosal stretch receptors whose output passes via sympathetic neurones to the central nervous system, while ulcers cause acid related pain mostly via vagal afferents.

Differential diagnosis

The commonest cause of anorexia, nausea, vomiting, and pain is duodenal ulcer disease, followed closely by functional

Figure 13.1 *Taking an emetic* by Isaac Cruickshank (1757-1810)

Table 13.1 Prevalence of symptoms in general population

Symptom	Frequency	Prevalence
Heartburn	>1/month	24%
	>1/week	13%
Upper abdominal pain	≥1/year	26%
	>6/year	16%
Acid regurgitation	>1/month	11%
	>1/week	7%
Upper abdominal pain lasting >2 hours		4%
Nausea	>1/month	8%
	>1/week	3%
Vomiting	>1/month	2%
Anorexia		4%
Weight loss >3 kg		3%

Table 13.2 Gastrointestinal symptoms in dyspepsia related diseases

% of patients with specified symptom

Symptom	FD	Oes	DU	GU	IBS	GS	ARD	GCa
Anorexia	40	35	47	56	35	29	55	64*
Nausea	39	17	34	39	32	28	37	48*
Vomiting	24	22	34	34	11*	23	59*	49
GI bleed	12	14	26*	23	5	7	32	34*
Heartburn	20	64*	32	23	12	19	25	22
Weight loss	23	20	26	34	16*	32	33	72
Psychotropic drug use	46*	35	26	20	38	31	18	9*

FD = functional dyspepsia, Oes = oesophagitis and reflux without oesophagitis, DU = duodenal ulcer, GU = gastric ulcer, IBS = irritable bowel syndrome, GS = gallstone disease, ARD = alcohol related dyspepsia, GCa = gastric cancer.
*Significant difference from other diseases

ABC of the Upper Gastrointestinal Tract

dyspepsia and irritable bowel syndrome. Gastric ulcer, gastro-oesophageal reflux, gastric cancer, and gall stones account for 5-10% each, and rarer diseases such as diverticular disease, small intestinal Crohn's disease, colon cancer, and pancreatitis make up the rest.

Pregnancy can, for a short while, be a mysterious cause of nausea and vomiting. Likewise, hepatitis during its prodrome, can be misleading, but the appearance of jaundice makes all clear. Even rarer are various metabolic diseases usually diagnosed in different contexts—such as diabetic ketoacidosis, renal tubular acidosis, and adrenocortical insufficiency—which may all present with anorexia, nausea, vomiting, and obscure abdominal pain.

The possibility of drug induced nausea should always be considered, especially with non-steroidal anti-inflammatory drugs, opiates, antibiotics, hormone preparations, and chemotherapeutic agents.

Limitations of gastrointestinal symptoms

Many studies have shown that diagnosis from individual gastrointestinal symptoms alone is difficult. Obviously different diseases do have a different spectrum of symptoms. Thus patients with gastric cancer frequently complain of profound anorexia, weight loss, and nausea while those with alcohol related dyspepsia typically vomit and retch especially first thing in the morning. Other differences that stand out include the frequent use of psychotropic drugs in functional dyspepsia and the high incidence of heartburn in oesophageal disease.

However, even seemingly serious indicators such as substantial weight loss (>3 kg), anorexia, and nausea are surprisingly common in functional dyspepsia, which, being so much commoner than gastric cancer, accounts for far more cases. Thus, most symptoms are neither specific nor sensitive for any particular condition. Even the classic features of peptic ulcer such as relief of pain by antacids or food and nocturnal pain, though commoner in peptic ulcer (65%, 75%, and 75% respectively) are sufficiently common in functional dyspepsia (60%, 40%, and 43% respectively) to be unhelpful in differential diagnosis.

One exception is perhaps biliary colic. This typically occurs in attacks with long periods of freedom from pain, which when it comes is located in the right upper quadrant and radiates to the tip of the shoulder. When pain comes on in the late evening, lasts over two hours, and is associated with sweating and vomiting then biliary colic is likely.

Demographic clues

Although symptoms are neither sensitive nor specific, including demographic details will improve matters. The ratio of organic to functional disease steadily increases with increasing age, since malignancy is very rare under the age of 45 (none in most case series), while the incidence of peptic ulcer increases linearly with age because of the increasing incidence of *H pylori* infection. Smoking is also associated with an increased risk of peptic ulcer and gastric cancer. Sex may also be a useful indicator: men are about twice as likely as women to have duodenal ulcer or gastric cancer, whereas women have a 50-60% increased risk of having irritable bowel syndrome and gallstone disease. Surprisingly, time taken off work from functional dyspepsia is as great or greater than it is from organic disease.

Non-gastointestinal features

Fortunately, distinguishing duodenal ulcer and functional dyspepsia, the two most likely causes, can be made easier by including more information about the patient. A history of

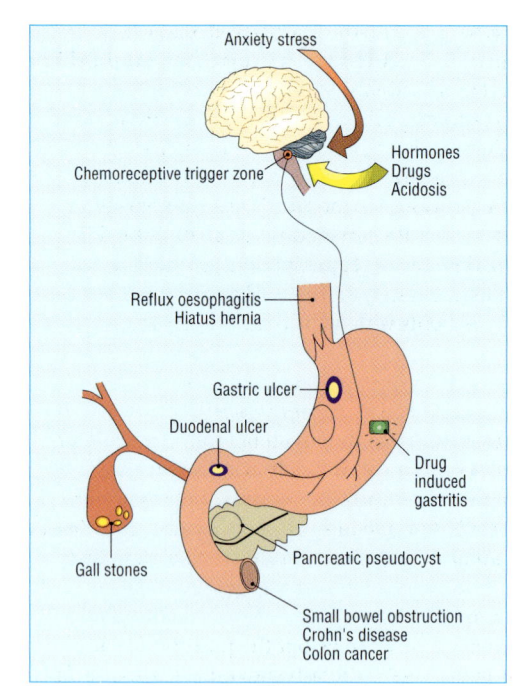

Figure 13.2 Possible reasons for anorexia, nausea, and vomiting with pain

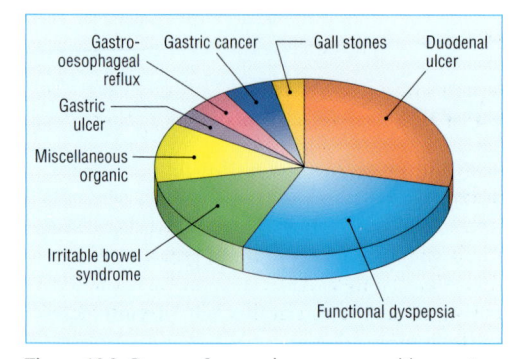

Figure 13.3 Causes of anorexia, nausea, vomiting, and gastrointestinal pain

Box 13.1 Metabolic causes of anorexia, nausea, or vomiting

- Diabetic ketoacidosis
- Renal tubular acidosis
- Hypercalcaemia
- Adrenocortical insufficiency
- Other rare causes of acidosis or alkalosis

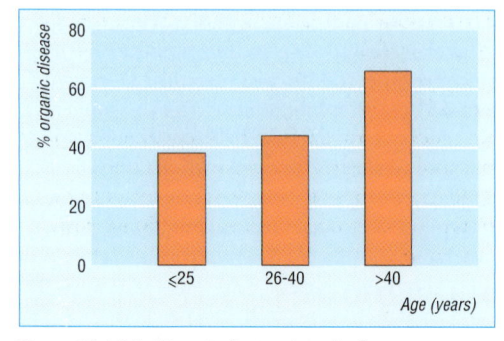

Figure 13.4 Likelihood of gastrointestinal symptoms being due to organic disease in different age groups

peptic ulcer is a strong predictor of further ulceration, while patients with functional dyspepsia score higher on depression and anxiety and tend to exhibit "somatisation."

Somatisation is characterised by recurrent multiple unrelated somatic complaints. They can be recognised by frequent visits to the doctor for many non-gastrointestinal disorders over the previous six months. These patients are more dissatisfied with their health care and perceive their health as poor. Exhaustion, time off work, palpitations, chest pain, breathing difficulties, and musculoskeletal symptoms are all more common in patients with functional dyspepsia.

H pylori status
H pylori infection, which can be reliably assessed from a urea breath test, is present in 90-95% of patients with peptic ulcer but in only 20-30% of those with functional dyspepsia. If *H pylori* status is combined with the psychosocial assessments mentioned above, 95% of patients with peptic ulcer and 80% of those with functional dyspepsia can be accurately identified.

Physical examination
Most examinations will be normal, but the presence of an abdominal mass or succussion splash suggesting obstruction of the gastric outlet is ominous and indicates the need for urgent referral, as does evidence of small bowel obstruction with abdominal distension and hyperactive bowel sounds.

Management

As always, this depends on a careful history and knowledge of a patient's medical and psychosocial background, together with his or her age.

Patients aged under 45
Given that malignant disease is very rare under the age of 45 years, it is reasonable to manage younger patients at initial presentation with a trial of either a prokinetic drug for nausea or an antisecretory agent for pain, together with appropriate advice about lifestyle.

If symptoms don't rapidly subside, however, they should be further investigated. Cost benefit analysis suggests that, although investigation is initially expensive, it increases patient satisfaction and is cheaper over the long term (>2 years) by reducing prescription costs and reconsultation rates. Testing for *H pylori* should be the first step, since a negative result allows one to exclude peptic ulcer with 90% confidence, provided that use of non-steroidal anti-inflammatory drugs is excluded.

Lifestyle adjustments such as weight reduction and avoidance of foods that aggravate symptoms will produce improvements in about half of patients, especially those with recent weight gain and heartburn.

A good response to a therapeutic trial of proton pump inhibitors supports a diagnosis of gastro-oesophageal reflux. Patients who fail to respond to treatment at this stage are likely to have functional dyspepsia.

Patients aged over 45
Since 66% of older patients are likely to have organic pathology, it is probably reasonable to refer all of them for further investigation, usually endoscopy. Testing for *H pylori* status is unlikely to be helpful in this group because infection is so common and hence non-specific.

After endoscopy
Endoscopy will give a specific diagnosis in 50-75% of cases. If symptoms occur in discrete attacks then ultrasound

---

Box 13.2 Key points in differential diagnosis of anorexia, nausea, and vomiting with abdominal pain

- Peptic ulcer is the commonest single cause
- >90% of patients with duodenal ulcer are infected with *H pylori*
- Functional dyspepsia, gastro-oesophageal reflux, and irritable bowel syndrome account for about half of cases
- Functional dyspepsia is characterised by frequent visits to doctor for non-gastrointestinal conditions, ingestion of psychotropic drugs, and negative *H pylori* status
- All patients aged >45 years with new symptoms lasting more than four weeks should be referred for investigation

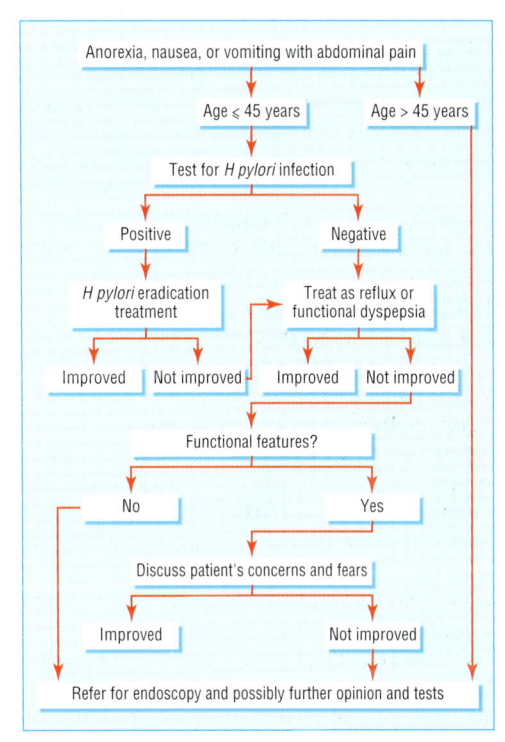

Figure 13.5 Algorithm for management of anorexia, nausea, vomiting, and pain

---

Box 13.3 Key points in management of anorexia, nausea, and vomiting with abdominal pain

Patients aged <45 years
- Persistent symptoms after a short trial of antisecretory or prokinetic drugs should be investigated by testing for *H pylori* infection
- Early investigation reduces prescription costs and repeat visits
- A negative test is as efficient as endoscopy in reassuring young patients that they do not have serious pathology

Patients aged >45 years
- Two thirds of patients will have organic pathology
- Early endoscopy is recommended
- Positive tests for *H pylori* infection are sensitive but not specific for peptic ulcer and hence of little value

investigation of the gall bladder should be considered. Otherwise, persistent symptoms in the absence of somatisation disorder warrant further investigation with barium follow through and computed tomography of the abdomen. If these fail to show any abnormality then functional dyspepsia is likely.

Functional dyspepsia
The most demanding, difficult patient who is never satisfied with your efforts is the most likely to have functional dyspepsia. Making the effort to uncover the underlying psychopathology may save many fruitless and elaborate tests. Active treatment of overt psychiatric disease or cognitive behavioural therapy with more limited aims may be appropriate for some patients.

Dyspepsia without obvious abnormality or somatisation
This should comprise a relatively small subgroup of patients for whom further investigations are indicated. Since endoscopy is relatively insensitive in diagnosing reflux, 24 hour oesophageal pH monitoring may be helpful. If pH monitoring is not available a therapeutic trial of proton pump inhibitors is a reasonable alternative and may produce a positive response in up to half of patients.

Other possibilities include delayed gastric emptying, which is seen almost exclusively in women. However, results from gastric emptying studies do not correlate well with symptoms so it is probably reasonable to give women with unexplained nausea and vomiting a trial of a prokinetic drug such as cisapride or metoclopramide without first undertaking such studies. Failing this, domperidone should be tried; this centrally acting dopamine blocker is inexpensive, well tolerated, and effective against nausea of central origin.

Box 13.4 Clinical summary
- Diagnosing the causes of anorexia, nausea, and vomiting depends on careful assessment of all the relevant features of patients' medical and drug histories together with physical examination
- Most patients are understandably anxious about the possibility of serious disease and will require some investigation
- Although duodenal ulcer is currently the commonest cause, it is declining and practitioners should be aware of the high incidence of functional dyspepsia in this setting
- By looking carefully for the signs of functional dyspepsia, doctors can make a positive diagnosis rather than one of exclusion after exhaustive and fruitless tests

Taking an emetic is reproduced with permission of the Wellcome Trust.

Index

Where not already indexed with a text reference, page numbers in **bold** refer to illustrations; those in *italic* to tabulated or boxed material

abdominal pain (upper)
   gall bladder 37–40
   nausea and vomiting with 45–8
achalasia 9, 11
   dysphagia caused by 12–13, 14, 15
acid perfusion test, in GORD 5, 10
acid reflux
   Barrett's oesophagus and 13
   dyspepsia and 1, 33
   dysphagia and 15
   upper abdominal pain 33
   see also gastro-oesophageal reflux
"acid" regurgitation, in GORD **4**
acid secretion, gastric 19–20
acid suppression therapy
   in NSAID-associated ulcers 27–8
   in oesophagitis 6–7
acute cholecystitis 37
acute upper gastrointestinal haemorrhage 30–2
adenocarcinoma
   dyspepsia in *33*
   gastric 41–2
      chronic atrophic pangastritis and 23
      dyspepsia and *33*
   oesophageal, risk of 6
   pancreatic 43
adrenaline injection, for non-variceal
      haemorrhage 32
aerophagy (air swallowing) 33, 36
age
   gastrointestinal haemorrhage and 30
   NSAID-associated ulcers 26–7, *27*
AIDS related oesophagitis, dysphagia in 15
air swallowing (aerophagy) 33, 36
"alarm" symptoms
   gastric cancer 34
   in GORD 5, *6*
alcohol-related disorders
   dyspepsia 46
   gastrointestinal haemorrhage 31
alendronic acid, peptic stricture and 13
alginates, for oesophagitis 6
amoxicillin, in low dose triple therapy 24, *25*
angina, upper abdominal pain 8, 9–10, *33*
anorexia 45–8
   in gastric cancer 41
antacids
   for dyspepsia 2
   for oesophagitis 6
anticoagulants, and NSAID-associated ulcers 27
antidepressants, for functional dyspepsia *36*
antioxidant vitamins (lack of), dietary factor in
      H pylori infection 21

antisecretory drugs
   for dyspepsia 2
   for functional dyspepsia *36*
   for gastric ulcer 23
   interactions between *H pylori* and GORD 23
antispasmodic agents, for functional dyspepsia *36*
antral gastritis 17, 20
anxiety
   achalasia 9, 11
   dyspepsia and nausea and vomiting **46**, 47
aortoduodenal fistula, haemorrhage and 31
aspirin
   gastrointestinal toxicity 26, *27*
   haemorrhage and 30
atrophic gastritis 23
autoimmune gastritis 17
azapropazone, gastrointestinal toxicity *27*

bacterial infection *see Helicobacter pylori*
balloon dilatation, gastro-oesophageal
      sphincter 11
barium radiology
   in chest pain 10
   in dysphagia 12
   in gastric cancer 41
   in GORD 5, *6*
   in nausea and vomiting 48
Barrett's oesophagus 5, 6, 7
   dysphagia caused by 13–14
   oesophageal cancer risk **23**
behavioural therapy, for functional
      dyspepsia *36*, 48
Bernstein test 8
beta-adrenoceptor blocker, in variceal
      haemorrhage 32
bile duct stones 37
   management 39
bile reflux 5
   and Barrett's oesophagus 13
bile salt dissolution therapy 39
bile salts, enterohepatic circulation 37, **38**
biliary colic *33*, 37
   characteristics of 34, 38, *38*, 46
biliary tract disease *33*
bismuth-based therapy
   for functional dyspepsia *36*
   for *H pylori* eradication 24
bloating, in dyspepsia 33, 34
blood group, and *H pylori* infection 21
botulinum toxin, for achalasia 11
bougies, for dysphagia 12
bowel ulceration, side-effect of NSAIDs 28
brachytherapy, for oesophageal tumours 14

Index

breath test, C-urea
  H pylori diagnosis 3, 18
  H pylori eradication and 22
bulbar palsy, dysphagia caused by *12*

CA 19.9, tumour marker 43
cagPI (pathogenicity island) strain, *H pylori* phenotype 21
calcium channel blockers, for oesophageal spasm 11
cancer *see* adenocarcinoma; carcinoma; gallbladder cancer; gastric cancer; gastrointestinal cancer; oesophageal tumours; pancreatic cancer
candida (monilial) oesophagitis, dysphagia in 15
carcinoembryonic antigen 43
carcinoma
  duodenal ulcer caused by **22**
  oesophageal 14
    Barrett's oesophagus and 13
    dysphagia caused by *12–13*
cardia, carcinoma of 12
cardiac pain, as upper abdominal pain 8, 9–10, *33*
cardiomyotomy, for achalasia *11*
celecoxib, COX-2 inhibitor **29**
chemotherapy
  in gastric cancer 42
  in oesophageal tumours 14
  in pancreatic cancer 44
chest pain
  cardiac 8, 9–10, *33*
  in GORD **4**
  oesophageal 8–11
cholangiography 39
cholecystectomy, laparoscopic 37, 39
cholecystitis, acute *37*
cholecystostomy 39
cholesterol stones 37
chronic atrophic pangastritis, and gastric cancer 23, 41
chronic pancreatitis, differential diagnosis 43
cigarette smoking 21, **24**, 27, 46
cimetidine, H₂ receptor antagonist 7
cineradiography, in dysphagia 12
cisapride, prokinetic drug 48
clarithromycin
  in low dose triple therapy 24, *24*, 25
  resistance to 24
CLO urease test, *H pylori* diagnosis 17–18
colitis, side-effect of NSAIDs *28*
computed tomography
  in nausea and vomiting 48
  in pancreatic cancer 42–3
"corkscrew oesophagus" 9
corpus gastritis 20
corrosive chemical ingestion, peptic stricture and 13
corticosteroids, and NSAID-associated ulcers 27
Courvoisier's law 43
COX-2 (cyclo-oxygenase-2 enzyme) inhibitors, new generation NSAID 29
cranial nerve palsy, dysphagia caused by *12*
cricopharyngeal spasm, dysphagia caused by *12*
Crohn's disease **19**, **22**
  gallstones and 37
  nausea and vomiting 46
culture, *H pylori* diagnosis 17, *18*
C-urea breath test
  H pylori diagnosis 3, 18
  H pylori eradication and 22

cyclo-oxygenase-2 enzyme (COX-2) inhibitors, NSAIDs 29
cytomegalovirus infection **22**

dental enamel erosion, in GORD **4**
depression and anxiety
  dyspepsia and nausea and vomiting **46**, 47
  oesophageal pain 9, 11
diabetes
  nausea and vomiting 46
  upper abdominal pain *33*
diclofenac, gastrointestinal toxicity 27
dietary factors, in *H pylori* infection 21
dietary fat
  gallstones and 37
  pancreatic cancer risk *43*
dietary modification, in dyspepsia 35
diflunisal, gastrointestinal toxicity 27
dilatation, gastro-oesophageal sphincter 11
diverticular disease, nausea and vomiting 46
domperidone
  for functional dyspepsia *36*
  for heartburn 7
  for nausea and vomiting 48
dopamine blocker, in nausea and vomiting 48
drugs
  dyspepsia caused by *35*
  nausea and vomiting caused by 46
  see also NSAIDs
drug treatments
  for gastrointestinal haemorrhage 32
  for NSAID-associated ulcers 27–8
duodenal ulcer 22
  gender and 46
  H pylori eradication and 25
  nausea and vomiting with 45–6
  pathophysiology 19–21
  side-effect of NSAIDs *28*
duodenogastric reflux 5
dyspepsia
  "alarm" symptoms *1*
  alcohol-related 46
  causes of 33–4
  functional *see* functional dyspepsia
  guidelines for investigation 42
  implications for the NHS 1–3
  management in primary care 2–3
  NSAID-associated 28–9
  symptoms *45*
dysphagia 12–15
  "alarm" symptoms 1, 5, *6*

ear, nose and throat symptoms, in GORD **4**
ectopic pancreatic tissue **22**
electrocoagulation, gastrointestinal haemorrhage 32
ELISA (enzyme-linked immunosorbent assay) antibody test 18
endoscopic retrograde cholangiopancreatography 43
endoscopy
  chest pain and 10
  cost/benefit of 1–3
  dyspepsia and 35
  dysphagia and 13–14
  gastric cancer and 41, **42**
  gastric ulcer and 23
  gastrointestinal haemorrhage 30, 31–2
  GORD and 5, *6*

Index

H pylori diagnosis 17
    nausea and vomiting and 47–8
enterochromaffin-like cells, in gastric acid secretion 19
epigastric pain 33
    gastric cancer and 41
    nausea and vomiting with 45–8
ethanolamine, sclerosant intravariceal injection 32
extracorporeal shock wave lithotripsy 39

faecal antigen test, *H pylori* diagnosis 18
famotidine, H_2 receptor antagonist 28
fenoprofen, gastrointestinal toxicity *27*
functional dyspepsia 24, 34–6
    acid secretion 19
    H pylori eradication and *25*
    nausea and vomiting in 45–6, 46–7, 48
fungal strictures, peptic 13

gallbladder
    cancer of 40
    impaired emptying and gallstone formation *37*, *38*
    upper abdominal pain 37–40
gall stones
    gender and 46
    management 39
    nausea and vomiting 46
    pain in *33*, 34
    risk factors *37*
gastrectomy 42
    pancreatic cancer risk *43*
gastric acid secretion, regulation 19–20
gastric cancer
    adenocarcinoma 41–2
        chronic atrophic pangastritis and 23
        dyspepsia in *33*
    "alarm" symptoms 34
    detection 3
    dyspepsia in 1, 34
    gender and 46
    H pylori and 16, 17, *25*
    nausea and vomiting 46
    pathophysiology 19–21
    prognosis 42
    risk factors *41*
    signs and symptoms *41*, 46
    treatment 42
gastric dysmotility, dyspepsia in **33**, 35, 36
gastric ulcer 23
    bleeding risk 23
    H pylori eradication *25*
    nausea and vomiting 46
    pathophysiology 19–21
    side-effect of NSAIDs *28*
gastrin, in gastric acid secretion 19
gastrin-secreting tumours 19, **22**
gastritis
    acid secretion and 20
    atrophic 23
    chemical **28**
    extent and location 20
    H pylori and 16, 17
gastroduodenal artery, erosion of 31
gastrointestinal cancer, haemorrhage and 31
gastrointestinal haemorrhage
    acute upper 30–2
    dyspepsia and *45*
    management 31–2
gastro-oesophageal reflux
    dysphagia caused by 12–13
    nausea and vomiting 46, 47
    predictors of 1
    see also acid reflux
gastro-oesophageal reflux disease (GORD) 4–7, 22, 23
    dyspepsia in 33
    H pylori and 23, *25*
gastro-oesophageal sphincter, balloon dilatation 11
gastrostomy, for dysphagia 12
G cells, in gastric acid secretion 19
globus hystericus 12
GORD *see* gastro-oesophageal reflux disease
granulomatous diseases, duodenal ulcer caused by **22**

H_2 receptor antagonists
    for duodenal ulcer 22
    for dyspepsia 2
    for functional dyspepsia 36, *36*
    for NSAID-associated ulcers 28
    for oesophagitis 6–7
haemorrhage *see* gastrointestinal haemorrhage
heartburn
    in dyspepsia 1, *45*
    in GORD 4–7, 33, 46
Helicobacter pylori
    acid secretion and 19–21
    asymptomatic 24
    diagnosis 16–18
        histology 17, *18*
        serology 3, 18
        stool antigen tests 3, 18
    dietary factors in 21
    dyspepsia and 3, 34
    epidemiology 16–18
    gastric cancer and 41
    GORD and 5–6, 23
    host factors 21
    management 22–5
        antisecretory drugs and 23
        eradication 24
            indications for *25*
            in NSAID-associated ulcers 28–9
    nausea and vomiting 46–7
    peptic ulcers and 23, 34
    phenotypes 21
Helicobacter pylori gastritis, in functional dyspepsia 34, 36
herpes simplex infection **22**
hiatus hernia **46**
    oesophagitis and 4–5
    pain in 33
histamine, in gastric acid secretion 19
hypercalcaemia
    duodenal ulcer caused by *22*
    upper abdominal pain *33*
hyperparathyroidism, duodenal ulcer and *19*
hypertensive ("nutcracker") oesophagus *9*

ibuprofen, gastrointestinal toxicity 27
indigestion
    definition 33
    NSAIDs and 26–9
indometacin, gastrointestinal toxicity *27*
irritable bowel syndrome
    biliary pain in 39

Index

irritable bowel syndrome – *Continued*
  dyspepsia in *33*, 35
  gender and 46
  nausea and vomiting with 45–6

jaundice
  gall stones and 38, 39
  nausea and vomiting 46
  pancreatic cancer and 43

ketoprofen, gastrointestinal toxicity 27

lansoprazole, proton pump inhibitor 7
laparoscopic anti-reflux surgery 7
laparoscopic cholecystectomy 37, 39
lecithin, in gallstone formation 37
leiomyoma **22**
leiomyosarcoma **22**
lithotripsy, extracorporeal shock wave 39
liver disease, gastrointestinal haemorrhage and 31
low dose triple therapy, *H pylori* eradication 24, 25
lymph node metastases, in gastric cancer 42
lymphoma **22**

malignant disease *see* adenocarcinoma; carcinoma; gallbladder
    cancer; gastric cancer; gastrointestinal cancer; oesophageal
    tumours; pancreatic cancer
Mallory-Weiss tears, gastrointestinal haemorrhage and 31
MALT lymphoma 25
manometry, in achalasia 15
mebeverine, antispasmodic agent *36*
meloxicam, new generation NSAID 29
mesenteric vascular insufficiency, upper abdominal pain *33*
metastases, in pancreatic cancer 42–3
metoclopramide
  for heartburn 7
  for nausea and vomiting 48
metronidazole, in low dose triple therapy 24, 25
migraine, sumatriptan cause of chest pain 9
Minnesota (Sengstaken-Blakemore) tube 32
misoprostol, prostaglandin E_1 analogue 27, 29
  for functional dyspepsia 36
monilial (candida) oesophagitis, dysphagia in 15
motility disorders
  gastric, dyspepsia in **33**, 35, 36
  oesophageal 8–11
  achalasia 15
motility modifying drugs, for oesophagitis 7
mucosal irritation, oesophageal 8
myasthenia gravis, dysphagia caused by *12*

naproxen
  gastrointestinal toxicity 27
  H pylori eradication and 28–9
nausea 45–8
  in gastric cancer 41
neoplasia, duodenal ulcer caused by *22*
NHS, cost of dyspepsia 1–3
nitrites, for oesophageal spasm 11
nitroimidazole antibiotics, resistance to 24
non-steroidal anti-inflammatory drugs *see* NSAIDS
non-variceal haemorrhage, treatment 32
NSAIDs
  gastrointestinal toxicity 26–7, *28*
    drug-induced nausea and vomiting 46
    drug-induced ulcers
      drug treatments for 27–8
      duodenal *19*, 22, 34
      gastric 23, 34
      H pylori eradication 25
  gastrointestinal haemorrhage 30–1
  indigestion 26–9
  peptic stricture 13
  use of 26
    management of 27
"nutcracker oesophagus" *9*

obesity, gallstones and 37
odynophagia 12
oesophageal band ligation 32
oesophageal manometry 10
oesophageal pH monitoring *see* pH monitoring
    (oesophageal)
oesophageal provocation tests 10–11
oesophageal tumours 14
  adenocarcinoma, dyspepsia in *33*
  cancer, dyspepsia in 1
  carcinoma, dysphagia caused by 12–13
oesophageal varices, haemorrhage and 31, 32
oesophagitis
  endoscopic findings **4**
  gastrointestinal haemorrhage and 31
  in GORD 4–7
  reflux 1, 33
  side-effect of NSAIDs *28*
oesophagogastrectomy 14
oesophagus
  chest pain 8–11
  "corkscrew oesophagus" 9
  dilatation for peptic stricture 13
  distention of 8–9
  heartburn and 4–7, 46
  motility disorders 8–11
    dysphagia caused by *12*
  "nutcracker oesophagus" 9
  rupture after dilatation 13, 15
  spasm 9, 11
    dysphagia in 15
  stricture **13**
    side-effect of NSAIDs *28*
  see also gastro-oesophageal reflux
omeprazole, proton pump inhibitor 7, 28, 29
  in triple therapy 25
oral contraceptive use, gallstones and 37
orophangeal malignancy, dysphagia caused by *12*

pain
  biliary colic 37, 38
  chest
    differential diagnosis 8–11
    in GORD **4**
  gastric cancer 41
  nocturnal 46
  retrosternal 1
    in hernia torsion 4
  upper abdominal 33
    cardiac 8, 9–10, *33*
    nausea and vomiting with 45–8
pain control
  in gastric cancer 42
  in pancreatic cancer 44
pain threshold, psychological factors 9

Index

palliative treatment
   in gastric cancer 42
   in pancreatic cancer 44
pancreatectomy procedures 44
pancreatic cancer 41, 43–4
   prognosis 44
   treatment 44
pancreatic pseudocyst **46**
pancreatitis
   chronic, differential diagnosis 43
   nausea and vomiting 46
   upper abdominal pain *33*
pangastritis 17
   Barrett's oesophagus and GORD and **23**
   chronic atrophic, and gastric cancer 23, 41
pantoprazole, proton pump inhibitor 7
parietal cells, in gastric acid secretion 19, 20
Parkinson's disease, dysphagia caused by *12*
patient counselling, in *H pylori* infection 24–5
peptic stricture
   dysphagia caused by 14
   postoperative 13
peptic ulcer 1–3
   dyspepsia in 1–3, 33–4
   haemorrhage and 30–1
   H pylori and 16, 17
   nausea and vomiting 46–7
   see also duodenal ulcer; gastric ulcer
periampullary tumours 43
pernicious anaemia 19, *41*
pharyngeal pouch, dysphagia caused by 12
pH monitoring (oesophageal) 5, *6*
   in acid reflx 8, 10
   in GORD 33
   in nausea and vomiting 48
pigment stones 37
piroxicam, gastrointestinal toxicity 27
polidoconal, sclerosant intravariceal injection 32
potassium supplements, peptic stricture and 13
pregnancy
   gallstones and 37
   nausea and vomiting 46
prokinetic drugs
   for functional dyspepsia 36
   for nausea and vomiting 48
propranolol, beta-adrenoceptor blocker,
      in variceal haemorrhage 32
prostaglandin E$_1$ analogue 27
proton pump inhibitors
   action of 19
   costs of 2
   for chest pain 10
   for duodenal ulcer 22
   for functional dyspepsia 36
   for nausea and vomiting 47
   for NSAID-associated ulcers 28
   for oesophagitis 6–7
   for peptic stricture 13
   in low dose triple therapy 24, 25
   interactions between *H pylori* and GORD 6, 23
psychological factors
   in achalasia 9, 11
   in chest pain 8, 9, 11
   in dyspepsia 35, 36
psychotherapy
   for functional dyspepsia 36
   for nausea and vomiting in functional
      dyspepsia 48
psychotropic drugs, in functional dyspepsia *45*, 46

quadruple therapy, *H pylori* eradication 24, **25**

radiology, in dysphagia 12
radiotherapy, for oesophageal tumours 14
ranitidine, H$_2$ receptor antagonist 7
ranitidine-bismuth-citrate, *H pylori* eradication 24
reflux, *see also* gastro-oesophageal reflux
reflux oesophagitis, pain in 33
reflux related dysmotility, dysphagia in 15
renal disorders
   nausea and vomiting 46
   upper abdominal pain *33*
respiratory symptoms, in GORD **4**
resuscitation, haemorrhage and 31
rofecoxib, COX-2 inhibitor **29**
rupture, after oesophageal dilatation 13, 15

salt, dietary factor in *H pylori* infection 21
sarcoidosis **22**
Schatzki's ring **13**
sclerosants, intravariceal injection 32
selective seretonin reuptake inhibitor *36*
Sengstaken-Blakemore (Minnesota) tube 32
serology, *H pylori* diagnosis 3, 18
smoking 21, **24**, **27**, 46
sodium tetradecyl sulphate, sclerosant intravariceal
      injection 32
somatisation, dyspepsia and nausea and vomiting **46**, 47
spasm, oesophageal 9, 11, 15
sphincter of Oddi, high pressure 39
stents, oesophageal 14
stomach
   cancer of 41–2
   oesophagogastrectomy 14
   see also gastric
stool antigen tests, *H pylori* diagnosis 3, 18
strictures
   oesophageal **4**, 7
   peptic 13, 14
stroke, dysphagia caused by 12
sucralfate, for functional dyspepsia 36
sulindac, gastrointestinal toxicity 27
sumatriptan, chest pain caused by 9
syphilis **22**

terlipressin, vasoactive drug 32
tolmetin, gastrointestinal toxicity 27
transjugular intrahepatic portosystemic
      shunt (TIPPS) 32
tricyclic antidepressants
   for achalasia 9, 11
   for functional dyspepsia *36*
Troisier's sign 41
tuberculosis **22**
tumour markers, in pancreatic cancer 43
tumours *see* adenocarcinoma; carcinoma; gallbladder
      cancer; gastric cancer; gastrointestinal cancer;
      oesophageal tumours; pancreatic cancer
tumours, duodenal ulcer caused by **22**

ulcer
   NSAID-associated 27–8, 28–9
   see also duodenal ulcer; gastric ulcer; peptic ulcer

Index

ultrasonography
  gall stone test 38
  in jaundice 43
upper abdominal pain
  gall bladder 37–40
  nausea and vomiting with 45–8
urea breath test, *H pylori* diagnosis 18
urease tests, *H pylori* diagnosis 17–18

vacuolating toxin (Vac A toxin), in *H pylori*
    phenotype 21

variceal haemorrhage, treatment 32
vasoactive drugs, gastrointestinal haemorrhage 32
vomiting 45–8
  in GORD **4**
  in hernia torsion 4

weight loss, in dyspepsia *45*, 46
Whipple's procedure 44

Zollinger-Ellison syndrome, gastrin-secreting
    tumour 19, **22**